# HIGHLIGHTS ON SEVERAL UNDERESTIMATED TOPICS IN PALLIATIVE CARE

Edited by **Marco Cascella**

**Highlights on Several Underestimated Topics in Palliative Care**
http://dx.doi.org/10.5772/63659
Edited by Marco Cascella

**Contributors**

Trisha Dunning, Masashi Kanai, Yu Uneno, Mitsuko Ushikubo, Cristina Endrizzi, Mirella Palella, Valeria Ghelleri, Roberta Bastita, Ger Wackers, Yaël Tibi-Levy, Martine Bungener, Padmashri Rastogi

**Published by InTech**

Janeza Trdine 9, 51000 Rijeka, Croatia



**Publishing Process Manager** Iva Lipovic
**Technical Editor** SPi Global
**Cover** InTech Design team

First published September, 2017
Printed in Croatia
Legal deposit, Croatia: National and University Library in Zagreb

Additional hard copies can be obtained from orders@intechopen.com

Highlights on Several Underestimated Topics in Palliative Care, Edited by Marco Cascella
p. cm.
Print ISBN 978-953-51-3565-4
Online ISBN 978-953-51-3566-1

For EU product safety concerns:
IN TECH d.o.o., Prolaz Marije Krucifikse Kozulić 3, 51000 Rijeka, Croatia,
info@intechopen.com or visit our website at intechopen.com.

# Meet the editor

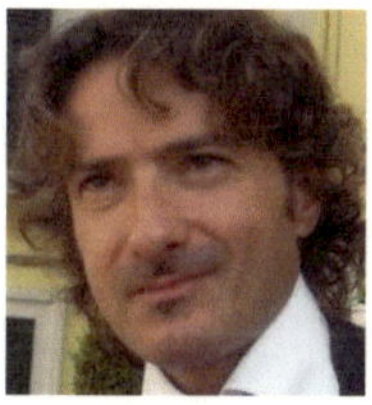

Marco Cascella, MD, PhD, works in the Department of Supportive Care at the National Cancer Institute, Fondazione "G. Pascale" – IRCCS, Naples, Italy, where he has responsibility for research in anesthesia and pain medicine. He is also Professor of Physiology on the Degree Course in Biomedical Laboratory Techniques at the Faculty of Medicine, University "Federico II", Naples, and Professor of Anesthesia, and Pneumology on the Degree Course of School of Nursing at the same University. Dr. Cascella graduated in Medicine and Surgery with honors, in 1997, at the Second University of Naples and then undertook postgraduate studies in anesthesia and intensive care, gaining his doctorate in 2001. Dr. Cascella acts as an editorial board member for several medical journals. He has been a speaker at numerous conferences and conventions, and is the author of about 80 scientific publications, books, book chapters, etc. in the fields of anesthesia, pathophysiology, treatment of pain, oncology, and palliative care.

# Contents

# Preface

This book does not intend to be a manual on palliative care and has not even been designed to offer an overview on a discipline which is very complex and difficult to talk about. On the contrary, this essay is a reflection on several topics which are too often underestimated in palliative care. Thus, it is devoted to special topics which have been identified after a careful examination of the latest medical literature on the subject.

The discussion is divided into four sections: Ethical Issues, Volunteers in Palliative Care, Special Circumstances and Prognostic Models in Palliative Care. Because Ethical Issues is a highly relevant basic theme of the matter, three chapters have been dedicated to it, and we enrolled in the authors' team international experts in the field. We are grateful to Prof. Endrizzi and associates, Padmashri Rastogi and Wackers Ger for their efforts. Any medical decision for a diagnostic or therapeutic decision mandates both a highly qualified indication, and the patient's consent as the patient himself is the expert of his life. We hope that this message can be well understood. For this purpose, the matter of the Early Integration of Palliative Care, the concepts of and Overdiagnosis and Overtreatment as well as the themes concerning the Balance sheets of suffering, Good Death, Euthanasia, Assisted suicide, and the question of the 'Do not attempt resuscitation' are exhaustively dealt.

Divided opinions concern the complex and controversial presence of non-professional actors such as Volunteers in Palliative Care. In their well-written chapter, Yaël Tibi-Lévy and Martine Bungener focused on the role of volunteers in France. They presented us an extensive overview of major issues of the topic also offering an interesting viewpoint of volunteers: "being there to be there". Maybe it represents the most detailed work on the subject.

Palliative Care has not been exhaustively focused on non-malignant diseases yet. The Special Circumstances addressed in this book are Diabetes and Amyotrophic Lateral Sclerosis. Diabetes is the most prevalent chronic disease. Consequently, in the chapter of Prof. Dunning Trisha, the reader is made aware that the management of diabetes and its complications is a significant issue to be addressed in palliative care settings in order to identify and manage diabetes-related symptoms and reduce health costs. On the other side, although Amyotrophic Lateral Sclerosis represents the most common degenerative disease of the motor neuron system, it has a significantly lower incidence than diabetes. Despite this, caring for individuals with Amyotrophic Lateral Sclerosis is a very hard task and needs to both start and end with palliative care in the physical, psychological, social, and spiritual aspects. In a dedicated chapter, Dr. Ushikubo addressed three unique characteristics of Amyotrophic Lateral Sclerosis care in Japan: the high level of disagreement between patients and family; the high rate of ventilator use compared with Western countries; and the low consumption of morphine.

In recent decades, many efforts have been made to develop Prognosis Prediction Models in Palliative Care. Their paramount role is to offer effective tools in order to facilitate optimal decision making for both physicians and patients. In his chapter, Dr. Masashi accurately reviewed the most commonly used prognosis prediction models in palliative care and related studies. In addition, he focused on their possible clinical utility and on the features of an ideal prognostic score.

The initial project of including further aspects of the discipline has been subsequently resized just to give more emphasis to few, but well-dealt with, pivotal topics. In addition, there was the risk of overlapping with the abundant editorial offer on the same topic. However, the four sections have been designed to be large containers. For instance, the topic Ethical Issues is not a complete topic at all whereas it is intuitive for those who work in palliative care that there may be an unprecedented number of Special Circumstances. Consequently, our aim is to gather suggestions and proposals (and also constructive criticisms) to plan subsequent book updates.

The authors hope that clinicians, nurses, volunteers and all the professionals involved in the management of the palliative care will find in this volume interesting reflections helpful for improving their daily work. Furthermore, the authors especially hope that students, resident trainees, and those who are facing the daily challenges of palliative care can find this volume useful in their very difficult but extraordinarily fascinating mission.

**Marco Cascella, MD, PhD**
Division of Anesthesia and Pain Medicine,
Istituto Nazionale Tumori – IRCCS – "Fondazione G. Pascale",
Naples, Italy

Section 1

# Ethical Issues

Chapter 1

# Reflection on Palliative Sedation for Existential Distress. It is Possible to Tolerate the Incomprehensible?

Cristina Endrizzi, Mirella Palella, Valeria Ghelleri and Roberta Bastita

Additional information is available at the end of the chapter

http://dx.doi.org/10.5772/intechopen.69860

**Abstract**

The difficulty of making decisions in end of life is the subject of these reflections through two clinical cases. We considered the question of palliative sedation for existential distress through a phenomenological approach, focusing the relationship between a patient's clinical history and the reactions of the care team to the existential distress of the patients. We chose to introduce a concept, dynamic projective identifications, which is a powerful mechanism for communication between human beings. The hypothesis is that projective identification works as a powerful mechanism of emotional contagion between people facing death, families, and their health workers. In the cases, however, the use of this therapeutic tool is not oriented to provide psychotherapeutic methods of supporting dying patients but to sustain the awareness of the care team in the decision-making process. The psychological pressure on the care team may lead physicians to act considering "what you already know". Being aware of these mechanisms can help physicians to understand the phenomena that are happening. Even if palliative sedation is the best therapy, the care team must clarify the meaning of the projective identification and enter them into the flow of communication with the patients and their families.

**Keywords:** palliative sedation terminal, existential distress, end-of-life making decision, projective identifications, death

## 1. Introduction

The confrontation with impending death triggers emotional reactions (e.g., feelings of grief, sadness, despair, anxiety, loss and loneliness, etc.), some of which are adaptive responses to preparatory grief [1]. Many patients are able to achieve acceptance of their illness and its prognosis, but each patient brings his/her own characteristic mode of coping and an array of strengths and vulnerabilities to the experience of a terminal illness. Systematic psychological assessment allows the clinician to support effective coping mechanisms and to identify persons at risk of experiencing high levels of difficulty during their illness [2]. Demoralization syndrome is an important clinical entity that is defined by the presence of pathological symptoms in the areas of mood, hope, and subjective competence. It is a personal experience of not coping with attacks on one's self efficacy and esteem [3]. In cancer patients, this process is sometimes described as "existential distress" [4], but it also occurs within the traditional psychiatric, and it is a risk factor for the manifestation of psychopathology. Demoralization is a spectrum that starts with subjective incompetence and non-pathological distress, and it can transition into helplessness, which sometimes grows into hopelessness. When it endures, it can be recognized as a syndrome that causes significant impairment in important areas of functioning [5]. Although some symptoms of demoralization are also expressed in existential distress at the end of life (feeling of apprehension, panic, threat, feeling of incompetence, of shame, impotence, aloneness, isolation, despair, etc.), existential distress manifests the experience of existential suffering in the context of an individual's confrontation with a specific stage of the dying process. Some people with certain personality traits, disadvantaged socioeconomic situations, or trauma histories in childhood might experience long-standing existential suffering (isolation, loss of dignity, meaninglessness, fear, etc.). Existential distress specifically develops as the result of facing one's impending death and is different from other reactions to end of life. In addition, existential distress must be distinguished from major depressive episodes, anxiety disorders, and delirium [6]. We refer to the definition article of Schuman-Olivier et al. ([7], p. 340) for definition and differential diagnosis from other psychiatric disorders. The authors have proposed a classification of existential distress based on the temporal context of the dying process: acute, subacute, and chronic are the general categories that focus on a person's proximity to likely death (imminent for acute and subacute, or <2 weeks, not imminent but life-threatening for chronic). We agree that the time available until death or loss functioning and a patient's baseline functional capacity to engage in the logistics of a therapeutic relationship are clear parameters to suggest therapeutic approaches (psychotherapy, psychopharmacological intervention up to palliative sedation) to clinicians and to help create a reliable decision-making language.

The questions of when and how to intervene with palliative sedation therapy (PST) are related to the concept of defining a refractory symptom [8]. Even if procedural guidelines for PST [9, 10] help physicians and care teams through the decision-making process and make them more comfortable to respond to physical sufferance, when their patients experienced any psychological symptom, physicians more frequently reported an emotional pressure [11]. Individual clinician bias, emotional exhaustion, or burnout can influence the decision-making process [12] as well as cultural, social, and ethical conditioning [13].

Therefore, the goal, on one hand, is to understand the peculiar suffering of patients (and their families) and, on the other hand, to analyze the psychological responses of the care team toward the suffering of a particular patient.

Through two narratives, we propose the physicians' work to comprehend the context (the patient's clinical history) in which the phenomenon of existential distress appears and make an effort to be aware of the projective identifications ([14], pp. 37–74). We refer to mostly raw emotion, which is unfiltered by the reflective function of thought, or proto-emotional and sensory elements [15] that bridge the relationship between the patient and the care provider (family, physicians, and care team).

The purpose of this contagion is that one can feel and experience what another person experiences, even bodily sensations and perceptions (embodiment), through a total affective communication process. If a care team is not trained to contain the projective identifications or is overwhelmed by them, it will likely unconsciously react, adding another disturbance to the patient, in what has been termed "projective counter identification" (in [14] p. 43, [16]).

Two cases are presented of hospice patients who manifest symptoms of existential distress during the last days of life. Because of the rapid progression of their diseases, it was not possible to identify a therapeutic space for the patients to undergo routine psychotherapeutic and psychosocial approaches that are useful for patients with advanced life-threatening illness. Both patients experienced acute and subacute existential distress. In these clinical examples, we highlight the importance of clarifying the projective identifications and entering them into the flow of communication with the health care providers not to make hasty decisions and to tolerate the wait to ensure understanding of each incoherent or bizarre phenomenon before defining it as a symptom requiring treatment. Particularly in cases in which it is difficult to establish the refractoriness of a symptom, or when PST seemed to be appropriate for psychological distress, the care team is helped by a psychological team to reflect and recognize PST as a potential "counterphobic defense to treat."

The authors have adopted a phenomenological approach to study the case focusing on the relationship between the clinical history elements (symptoms, reaction to changes in therapy, biographical context, emotional, and behavioral relationships with significant others) and the countertransference reactions of care teams.

The countertransference refers in these cases to the use of emotions, images, thoughts, etc., within the care team, that are stimulated by what the patient and family live and feel [17, 18]. The survey method is qualitative and descriptive. Objective parameters (vital signs, pain and other symptoms, etc.) are noted in the diary, as well as the steps of the decision-making process, described in narrative form from the interviews with the patient and family.

The hospice team has a psychologist who specializes in psycho-oncology and three physicians with experience in palliative care. One of the physicians has also been a dance movement therapist since 2006 and a psychotherapist with training in expressive therapies. She is the narrator of the case histories reported here. The narrative approach is one method of revealing the intensity of end-of-life meetings and developing awareness reflection [19].

In these cases, the focus was on observing the events from a medical point of view, with precise job roles within the care team (i.e., observing from the perspective of "from the inside"), as well as observing through psychotherapy instruments and nonverbal language, thereby stimulating the support and elaboration of the "*thinking functions*" ([20], pp. 61–79) "on the edge" of the team. These narratives are reported in the context of the work team, with the supervision of the psychologist, to discuss the suitability of PST.

## 2. Clinical cases

### 2.1. Albert

An anonymous patient referred to as "Albert" was a 56-year-old male, married with a young daughter and an adopted adult child from a previous marriage. He was described by friends as a brilliant, educated, and intelligent man who was a consummate reader. His wife told us that he referred to himself as rational and lacking affection, unable to handle emotions, with cultivated areas of rewarding personal interest not shared with his family. He was well informed of his terminally illness (a progression of prostatic cancer with secondary bone lesions) and was admitted to hospice after an episode of major depression and a suicide attempt.

At the time of admission, the patient had urinary incontinence, the inability to walk and postural instability. He became dependent for all daily activities. The patient was extremely anxious and frightened by the pain, as well as feeling like a burden to his family and losing control of his own autonomy. He said that he was worried that when he died, his wife would not be able to provide for his daughter "as she should."

We started specific therapy to address his pain and antidepressants, with some initial benefit. However, the episodes of pain occurred more frequently, as did his anxiety, despite changes to the therapy (**Figure 1**).

The patient was in despair, and he wished to die. Facing refractory pain and anguish, we spoke with him about "conscious" or mild palliative sedation and the option of receiving additional doses of sedatives (intermittent sedation) when he desired to sleep. This proposal seemed to reassure him, perhaps returning to the patient the opportunity to regain some control by managing his symptoms. His wife took part in this conversation. She remained still and silent, sitting in the middle of a chair away from her husband's bed. Outside the room, she told us that the patient had repeatedly asked for euthanasia and that she disagreed with the mild or conscious sedation, as this option would not have protected her husband from the awareness of death. Confronted with oscillating sedation, in which the patient retained moments of awareness or reacted to surrounding stimuli, she showed apprehension and insisted that the sedation should be continuous and deep.

The patient spent nearly 20 days starting to again read and receive friends. He ate with an appetite and agreed to mobilize in a wheelchair, even going out for small trips. To the staff, he seemed to be sensitive and empathetic; however, his behavior with his wife seemed distant and not affectionate. I met him every day for visits with conversations about his tales of life.

http://dx.doi.org/10.5772/intechopen.69860

| Recovery days | Symptoms | Drugs (dosage/day) | Follow-up |
|---|---|---|---|
| Prehospitalization | Major depression | Duloxetine 60 mg<br>Olanzapine 15 mg (in three divided doses)<br>Alprazolam 0.75 mg (in three divided doses) | Antidepressant therapy was not changed until the week before his death |
| | Neuropathic pain from spinal metastases | Naropin 150 mg + Morphine hydrochloride 6 mg for peridural by elastomeric infusion device<br>Naropin peridural bolus 5 mg as needed<br>Transmucosal fentanyl (tm) 400 μg need to be administered<br>Morphine hydrochloride 10 mg for subcutaneously injection) | Necessary amendments to pain killers |
| First 3 days | Neuropathic pain<br>Numerical Rating Scale (NRS) 6/7<br>More than three episodes/day with NRS > 8 | Naropin 150 mg + Morphine hydrochloride 6 mg for peridural by elastomeric infusion device<br>More than 800 micr Fentanyl tm<br>At least 10 mg Morphine hydrochloride for subcutaneous injection<br>At least 20 mg of Naropin for peridural catheter divided into four boluses | Episodes of intense pain; effectively addressed by parenteral morphine (NRS from 10 to 4)<br>Changes in sensation and voluntary movement of the lower limbs |
| | Crisis of anxiety associated with pain, insomnia, and agitation | Midazolam 10 mg for subcutaneous injection as needed (at least two doses during the night) | When awake thoughts are fixed on the pain with an anticipatory anxious attitude |
| From 4 to 24 days | Neuropathic pain<br>Side effects of an overdose of anesthetic via epidural<br>The patient spoke of problems in life and expressed a wish to die; returning to thoughts of suicide<br>Asked to be euthanized<br>Faced the possibility of a palliative sedation with the addition of a benzodiazepine (Midazolam) by continuous infusion at doses that do not induce awareness reduction<br>Patient managed his sedation "on demand" | Added dexamethasone 8 mg for intravenous infusion<br>Elastomer suspended by epidural; small amount of naropine by epidural (from 150 to 80 mg) with four boluses of 20 mg every 12 h during the day<br>Elastomer device intravenous (Morphine hydrochloride 50 mg + 15 mg Midazolam)<br>Midazolam 20 mg in 250 ml saline at 20 ml/hour for hypnotic purposes | The patient returned to reading, receiving friends, resting all night, eating at the table, and walking about the room<br>Pain control requires periodic adjustments of doses of intravenously infused drugs |

| Recovery days | Symptoms | Drugs (dosage/day) | Follow-up |
|---|---|---|---|
| From 24 to 33 days | Leakage of the epidural catheter and accentuation of pain<br>Neurological side effects increasing opioid and benzodiazepine (concentration deficits, ideomotor slowdown, and impairment of concentration) | Increased dosage of morphine hydrochloride in 90 and 60 mg of midazolam in elastomeric device intravenous<br>Dexamethasone was reduced from 8 to 4 mg | Ideomotor slowdown with lucid and coherent; ataxia with postural instability in standing position. Able to receive visits, talk, listen to music but finds it impossible to read<br>A week before death reported having seen *Out of body experience* |
| From 34 to 39 days | Total pain with a prevalence of existential pain<br>Reported desperation because the contact with reality was slipping<br>The patient was reassured not to be afraid of his dreams and imagination<br>In the end, we proposed a continuous sedation | Morphine hydrochloride 120 mg and midazolam 90 and 100 mg chlorpromazine into elastomer device intravenously<br>Haloperidol 6 mg divided into three doses | Sedation oscillated at times the patient responds to verbal stimuli or to the presence of people, and when he awakens takes water and/or semi-soft food<br>Refers to hearing death approaching |

**Figure 1.**

Once, we used expressive therapy to represent his emotions and thoughts. I invited his wife to stay, but she preferred to leave.

I felt discomfort between the couple, although I did not understand why. I think that his wife left out of respect for his privacy perhaps as she used to. Albert insinuated that his wife did not want to participate because he had always demonstrated little emotion with her. He seemed sorry for this situation, and I thought that there was a sense of unworthiness and mortification, as it had appeared after the interview with the psychologist.

We drew on the same sheet, just like playing chess, his favorite game. We noted the difference in our traces. His was rigorous and linear, crossing the sheet directly. My trace ran under his and sometimes outlined a colorful space.

He said: "It's wonderful that you colour inside my lines." He found that one of the colored spaces seemed like Fonzie's hair tuft. We joked about this because Albert was left bald after chemotherapy. I thought that an element of narcissistic gratification could have been present. Despite the tone, the dialogue was lighter and less desperate. Albert talked about his own death and his wish to die (WTD). To end was no longer seen as an affront or undignified, and he no longer experienced the loss of control in making decisions. He would have shown his family how one can die, as a way of instructing them and giving them time to deal with the loss.

By the 18th day of hospitalization, Albert reported proprioceptive changes before waking up (e.g., one leg was larger than the other, his mouth was smaller, or one-half of the body slid diagonally in space). He spoke about these phenomena as an attentive witness. He understood his detachment from reality as a sign of impending death. The patient did not ask for a reduction of consciousness, even when he was in despair. Despite oscillating between drowsiness and wakefulness, he retained an awareness of death and dying until a few days before his death, when continued palliative sedation was initiated at his request. After Albert's death, I talked with his wife once again to ask permission to report this story. On that occasion, I had the opportunity to make my unease at the request for euthanasia known to her and told her that the mild and respite sedation had given Albert an opportunity to be together with his family and friends. Laconically, turning her head slightly sideways and with a smile she said something that I do not remember exactly but it could sound something like, "I would have preferred euthanasia."

### 2.2. Discussion of Albert's case

In this case, the care team is involved in different perspectives.

From the psychological point of view, the care team felt a sense of inadequacy and impotence toward the patient's wife, who insistently demanded deep sedation. Health workers were conflicted by the emotional pressure of his wife's, although the pharmacological treatment had ameliorated the quality of life of the patient, that started to eat, to receive friends, to read again and he agreed to mobilize in a wheelchair, with a sort of resilience, nonetheless in a difficult condition. Albert talked about his own death and his wish to die in a way less desperately. It seemed to emerge a new significance of his death, with a sort of project brought out: he would have shown his family how one could die, as a way of instructing them and giving them time to deal with the loss. The care team felt inspired from image behind the expression "You colour inside my lines" that Albert said at the end of expressive encounter with artistic material supporting the verbal dialogue. Albert manifested a capacity to be ironic about the changes of body image that is intrinsically linked to identity and the meaning of dignity [21]. Through the pharmacological treatment, the attention and the listening, the care team had returned to Albert the control of his end-of-life decision, prevented by burdening of symptom's disease and psychological distress.

The care team struggled with the request of euthanasia; therefore, the second point of analysis has been from this perspective. Albert represented cases in which a wish to die (WTD) persists even if pain is treated in a palliative care model [22]. A desire to hasten death is associated with functional impairment related to pain, and, moreover, it is a measure of pain severity in some studies [23]. Therefore, the significant decline in pain intensity levels was not predictive of an improvement in the desire to hasten death, particularly in patients in the last days of life, for whom other symptoms may also be associated with psychological distress, such as depression with insecure attachment, low self-esteem, and younger age [24]. Probably for these reasons, the patient's wife insisted with the therapy addressed to the abolition of consciousness (instead of the euthanasia, not legally performed in Italy). The care team, in line with the emotions and embarrassment expressed in the narrative explicit above and experienced by the physician in the encounters with the patient, referred the sense of unworthiness and mortification felt in the room when the wife was into a low self-esteem relationship or to reactualization in the couple of an insecure attachment. We have no other data on past to support this analysis, but the possibility *"to colour the lines inside of mine,"* recalled a new chance for Albert to experience himself in the relationship with the care team, instead of a crystallized, fixed and "black and white" defenses.

After all, WTD is a complex subjective and social phenomenon, a process rather than a mental state, in which it is important to explore not only the reasons or triggering factors, which can be treated, but also how a WTD makes sense for the patients [25]. Caregivers have a great responsibility because the WTD can be influenced by conversations about them. Then, to cultivate the skill of active listening, to reflect on their own ideas and fears about death, and to facilitate the patient's inner dialogue and discussion of his/her wishes about life and dying are the tasks required to assist patients in formulating their connection to their personal values and perspectives [26].

At this point, the care team had clarified that the request of the patient's wife could not be accepted as a surrogate decision, and the woman must be helped to tolerate the process of awareness of patient in front of his death. Nevertheless, the care team needed to tolerate the insistent demand of the wife, highlighting the ability of Albert to be the main interlocutor of end-of-life decisions and understanding that the psychological pressure experienced by the care team (that is the result of a projective identification) was attuned with the anxiety of the woman overwhelmed by the proximity of the death (in the context of the psychological and relational dynamics experienced in the couple, understood only partially). The PST could be the best chance, but the way and the time should be arranged with the patient.

Now we face with the third perspective of analysis. How should we interpret the proprioceptive impairment that occurred near the death? Was it a sign of delirium? If this hypothesis was correct, how we should consider the patient, competent or not competent?

The patient had, as we have shown in **Figure 1**, a complex drug therapy and a high-dose of neuroleptic drugs. There are insufficient clinical studies that allow one to clearly determine whether certain patient expressions that could be considered bizarre or incoherent are attributable to drugs with known neurological side effects or to impairment of thought function (e.g., delirium at the end of life) or whether they belong to a degree of consciousness that is part of the process of preparing for death.

The recent information available on proprioception suggests the role of small-diameter sensory cortical fibers representing each body part. For example, immediate distortion of body size with local anesthesia has been linked to loss of input from small-diameter fibers [27]. Findings in cardiac arrest survivors suggest that central hypercapnia and peripheral hypoxia, secondary to cerebral ischemia, cause a cortical hyper-activation that helps to explain the phenomenon of increased awareness in these patients in the absence of cerebral activity [28]. On the other hand, the cerebral ischemia is responsible for metabolic alterations also involved in nociceptive synaptic transmission, such as the inhibition of the production of nitric oxide, a free radical that regulates the cerebral phenomena of apoptosis. It would seem that it was implicated in the long-term potentiation (LTP), which supports the reinforcement of the synaptic transmission of spinal neurons and in fact represents an expression of a memory of the nociceptive stimuli [29, 30]. It is also known that pharmacological interventions can change the function of nociceptive neurons by transforming them into broad spectrum neurons of potential action (wide dynamic range or WDR) that receive impulses not only from the nociceptive system but also through the sense of touch and heat, which leads one to assume a link between nociception and proprioception, particularly in situations of peripheral or central hypersensitivity [31].

Therefore, the care team pointed out some questions: this phenomenon should be understood in the contest of the peripheral desensitization induced by drugs that act on mu receptors and GABA receptors (such as the association opioids and benzodiazepines) or as a cortical hyperactivation that occurs in the phenomena of near-death experience? Was it possible that Morphine and Midazolam hydrochloride in high doses act like a block anesthetic causing distortions in body size (like the proprioceptive alteration of Albert)? What was the relationship between the cortical areas of expansion representing the body parts and more complex alteration of body image in people who are dying taking neuroleptic drugs?

Thus, it was difficult to conclude whether the described phenomenon of depersonalization could be understood in the context of existential distress or if it has been caused by a pharmacological effect or a more complex alteration of body image in people who are dying. Some authors believe that the process of dying may consist of the translation of a progressive withdrawal of psychic energy in the neurological and peripheral nervous systems [32, 33]. The importance of defining this phenomenon was related to determining a strategy to treat it (pharmacological treatment up to palliative terminal sedation, or other approaches as psychotherapy, touch therapy, etc.).

Eventually, we regarded to this proprioceptive impairment like a sign of the disorder of the "body-container" [34] that could be a cause of anguish and could also explain the manifestation of proprioceptive reactions that often occur in a seriously ill patient [35]. Clinging to objects, fear during passive mobilization in bed, increased muscle tension, motor restlessness secondary to the loss of bowel control or failure to deplete the elimination organs such as the bladder and rectum, and the lack of perception of body parts could be an expression of primitive anguish. In the case of Albert, changes in proprioception had been integrated with vestibular afferents and condensed in the content of "dream thought" in the form of imagination, visions, and hallucinations. Although drugs administered may account for a cognitive dysfunction, it is interesting to note that hallucinations were concomitant to the general decay of the patient and were present close to death after a relatively long period of therapy, which still ensured a good quality of life. What was interesting in this case was that the presumed hallucinations of the patient were only of a kinesthetic nature, and this aspect was contextualized in the attitude of a person with difficulties making body contact.

We considered Albert competent and aware of the death impending, therefore we accepted his ability to let us known the proper time to start unconsciousness sedation.

### 2.3. Edy

Edy was an anonymous name for a 73-year-old married woman, with two sons and a husband. She suffered from dilated cardiomyopathy. For many years, Edy faced her cancer diagnosis and chemotherapy with a type of awareness that was obscured by an unjustified expectation of healing. Cancer of the rectum was already in an advanced stage, with liver metastases and infiltration of the uterus—at the time of diagnosis, 6 years to our knowledge. Edy had faced surgery and chemotherapy, apparently delegating her husband to receive information about the evolution of the clinical oncology. In fact, Edy unconsciously led her husband to believe what she wanted to believe, thereby causing him to downplay or cast doubt on the information received. Her husband had some type of dissociation from the information that he received. He seemed to be aware, though he had an emotional reaction of denial or devaluation (the same reaction demonstrated by his wife). Therefore, in terms of communication, the couple seemed to function as a unique individual.

Within a year, there were sub-occlusive symptoms, with two hospitalizations for nausea, vomiting, and lack of canalization of the intestine, which appeared to show peritoneal carcinomatosis.

We met Edy at her home, after she had started palliative home care on the advice of her oncologist, who intended to reduce hospital admissions for clinical symptoms by utilizing only symptomatic treatment. The husband was visibly fatigued and short of breath, but he was bustling around his wife and received us in the living room.

The logistical setting did not seem to function well for their needs. The bedroom was likely located on the top floor of the house, which was accessed through a staircase, with no handrail. In the room, there were two leather sofas. It resembled a showroom (visible but not touchable). The husband offered us two chairs in front of Edy, who was sitting at the dining table. The chairs were solid wood and uncomfortable. It was difficult to imagine that Edy could remain sitting there for very long. The conversation was dry. The symptoms that we were supposed to be treating were discussed openly, but we were warned that many good, reliable doctors (whose advice, we thought, could not be discussed) were attending to the family, including the family doctor, physical therapist, and cardiologist (who treated Edy's husband, as well as Edy's atrial fibrillation). Indeed, it seemed that only the cardiological therapy was the most important, because it was "life-saving." The examination of the patient did not indicate an acute phase diagnosis, although there was diarrhea indicative of a sub-occlusion, but the treatments that we had prescribed were stopped by the patient with advice of her family, as soon as we left the house.

A few days later, we received a phone call notifying us that the patient had been admitted to Oncology Department again. Another 15 days passed, and the patient was then transferred to hospice. Edy then appeared to be depressed and tired; however, her sons insisted on moving their mother to an armchair. When Edy refused food, they urged her to eat. Edy's husband was taciturn and present only when one of the sons was with him; he never asked us for information, and sometimes, he did not visit his wife for an entire day. Edy seemed to have chosen him as the subject toward whom to express her anger.

She also showed a certain level of contempt toward us. She snapped bitterly at the health workers who helped her with her basic needs. With her husband, she would let loose. However, this behavior did not seem to disturb the family.

There was a tendency to "normalize" everything in the family and not interpret Edy's unfriendly and rejecting manners as an aspect of her anger and mortification.

Her adult children refused to accept the recommended psychological support. However, it finally emerged through the sons that there was a possibility that Edy felt betrayed by her family because they had given up on bringing her home. This admission in hospice provided a way for Edy of dealing with topics, such as disappointment, the rupture that she sensed with the world, and the likelihood that her autonomy was irretrievably lost.

We had already prescribed antidepressants. We were witnesses to not only the physical decay of her body but also a particular manner of rejecting the world and preparing for death, which was also a source of anxiety for the team.

Edy became silent, without conditions or compromises. We tried various relational approaches, but there was no longer a productive relationship for an alliance with the patient regarding her decisions and desires. We tried to talk to her about the possibility of using a sedative type rescue dose, to discontinue the "passive" waking moments, but the patient, with her eyes closed, denied us even eye contact, saying, "I sleep enough already." We felt cornered, closed in and somehow gagged. When performing hygienic care in the morning, providing treatment or administering medication, some of the team members felt crushed by the silence and the passivity of the patient. The health care professionals were competing to stimulate or to induce Edy to answer merely yes or no.

We seemed to have become lost in the same trap that her sons were in: trying to please her, to stimulate her, or to talk to her in the belief that she could hear. It was strange that in front of her motionless body and her calm breathing, as if sleeping, with her muscle tone flabby from passive mobilization, that no one would think that she might have been in a state of coma. Everyone continued in the belief that she could understand what we were saying but that she wanted to punish us with her silence. We examined her again, excluding a state of coma. The feelings of alienation, depersonalization, and derealization that we felt when facing Edy not only excluded us from her world but also effaced us. From this perspective, we understood the reactions of the family members when faced with the proposal of respite sedation: "No, because it would extinguish her completely."

Clearly, it was a fact with which we did not agree; however, we could not overlook it. We did not have the support of the patient or her family members. In some last words spoken by Edy in the 15 days before her death, she told a nurse, "Here I am committing suicide." The tense used in the sentence referred to an action that was in progress, so the nurse thought she was dreaming in real time. However, following questions by the nurse, Edy replied, "I'm not dreaming, it is precisely what is happening; see, I'm committing suicide."

### 2.4. Discussion of Edy's case

In this case, the burden on the family in end-of-life decisions is clear, as was how little attention is still given to the process of awareness of the disease and poor prognosis before arriving at the point of palliative care [36]. The demand for information is not uniform in our society, and the role played by the families of terminally patients and in the attitude of physicians toward information disclosure clearly differs from the Northern European or Anglo-Saxon model [37]. Sometimes, the problem is how to inform a patient who is not willing to be informed. The culturally established *modus operandi* obliges the health care professional to be discrete when discussing cancer [38]. Moreover, the patient is free to use their autonomy even to delegate. The patient must decide how much autonomy he or she wishes to exercise, and this amount likely varies from culture to culture. In addition, many families are opposed to inform the patients of their conditions [39] as demonstrated by the second case, such cases can evolve and become difficult to treat. It is obvious that these are situations in which the team feels guilty about a shortcoming, something that could have been done or that they were not doing. As care providers, we are not satisfied with these cases, but we have to accept that this individual had long eluded her diagnosis and had experienced the disease as if it concerned another person, forcing those around her to feel that her anger was directed precisely toward herself, and she wanted the world to experience a sense of guilt. It may be possible that in cases in which a person is alienated from the awareness of death, there must be an extreme effort of self-denial and self-punishment to break away from the body, as in the case of Edy. In addition, in the conflict between family and care providers, palliative sedation for existential distress, even if appropriate, could not have been of benefit because it could cause further distress. Therefore, the dramatic sentence repeated to the nurse by Edy "I'm committing suicide" talks about not an intention but probably resumed the psychic dynamics in the relational field.

With her mutism, Edy elicited in the caregivers (care team and family) a feeling of impotence; with the refuse to eat elicited a sense of guilty; when she was acting out a state of coma, caregivers thought that she could understand what we were saying but that she wanted to punish us with her silence. With this passive attitude, the care team was obliged to feel her alienation and depersonalization. But like her family, the care team did not understand this powerful mechanism of psychic contamination; in front of anger, fear, and anguish of the patient, it could not find a way to deal with the subject of the imminent death and so doing, was allied to the defense mechanisms of the family (untruth, avoidance, and the complaisance, trying to please her or to stimulate her).

The care team countertransference seemed to be that it was expressed by the family when PST was proposed "the feeling that the doctors killed a loved one." The sentence of Edy about committing suicide reverses the roles, attributing to herself the damaging action (that caregivers attribute to themselves). In this sentence, Edy became in certain way assertive again and self-determined (in the sentences she is able to act), while the care team, with regret, could see mirrored its inability to propose their active role (the dialogue for truth, the support to the patient's role in end-of-life decision).

## 3. Conclusion

Sometimes troubled relationships that are full of emotions will short-circuit between the patient, family, and care team when they are inexorably facing the possibility of death and, sometimes, sudden death, during the process of a rapidly advancing, progressive, serious illness. The knowledge of some powerful mechanisms of communication, such as projective identifications, can explain the intensity of emotional involvement and the difficulty in making important decisions. Knowledge of this mechanism can become an instrument (as in psychodynamic psychotherapy and psychoanalysis) to understand what happens to a person who is living an end-of-life experience and to help health care professionals tolerate conflicts that overshadow important clinical decisions. In such cases, the guidelines that establish the decision-making process in these areas of care, although useful, are not sufficient to guide choices and decisions shared between the team and family. Both cases are suitable for PST, but in the first case, the problem was tolerating the wife's requests for deep sedation, which did not align with the patient's dissociative phenomena and persistent WTD; in the second case, the PST that seemed to be appropriate (because of the existential distress that was strongly expressed) was not achieved due to the family conflicts and poor auto-determination of the patient, who was not cognitively impaired. The care team, who had to share and develop intense feelings of frustration and doubt, also had to, at minimum, not surrender to an analysis based on "what you already know." It is known that in care team, this psychological pressure might result in physicians acting inappropriately [40, 41] before considering the need to understand the meaning of what is being observed. We agree that more training needs to be provided to physicians and palliative care teams [42].

## Author details

Cristina Endrizzi*, Mirella Palella, Valeria Ghelleri and Roberta Bastita

*Address all correspondence to: c.endrix@alice.it

Hospice Il Gelso, ASL Al, Piedmont, Italy

## References

[1] Periyakoil VS, Noda AM, Kraemer HC. Assessment of factors influencing preservation of dignity at life's end: Creation and the cross-cultural validation of the preservation dignity card-sort tool. Journal of Palliative Medicine. 2010;13:495-500. DOI: 10.1089/jpm.2009.0279

[2] Miovic M, Bloch S. Psychiatric disorders in advanced cancer. Cancer. 2007;15:1665-1676. DOI: 10.1002/cncr.22980

[3] Clarke DM, Kissane DW. Demoralization: Its phenomenology and importance. Australian and New Zealand Journal of Psychiatry. 2002;36:733-742. DOI: 10.1046/j.1440-1614.2002.01086.x

[4] Kissane DW. Psychospiritual and existential distress: A challenge for palliative care. Australian Family Physician. 2000;29:1022-1025

[5] de Figueiredo JM. Distress, demoralization and psychopathology: Diagnostic boundaries. European Journal of Psychiatry. 2013;1:61-73. https://dx.doi.org/10.4321/S0213-61632013000100008

[6] Crunkilton DD, Rubins VD. Psychological distress in end-of-life care: A review of issues in assessment and treatment. Journal of Social Work in End-of-Life & Palliative Care. 2009;5(1-2):75-93. https://dx.doi.org/10.1080/15524250903173918

[7] Schuman-Olivier Z, Brendel DH, Forstein M, Price BH. The use of palliative sedation for existential distress: A psychiatric perspective. Harvard Review of Psychiatry. 2008;16(6):339-351. DOI: 10.1080/10673220802576917

[8] Bruera E. Palliative sedation: When and how. Journal of Clinical Oncology, Commentary. 2012;30(12):1258-1259. DOI: 10.1200/JCO.2011.41.1223

[9] Cherny N, Radbruch L. European Association for Palliative Care (EAPC) recommended frame work for the use of sedation in palliative care. Palliative Medicine. 2009;23(7):581-593. DOI: 10.1177/0269216309107024

[10] Kirk TW, Mahon M. National Hospice and Palliative Care Organization (NHPCO) position statement and commentary on the use of palliative sedation in imminently dying terminally ill patients. Journal of Pain and Symptom Management. 2010;39(5):914-923. DOI: 10.1016/j.jpainsymman.2010.01.009

[11] Blanker MH, Koerhius-Roessink M, Swart SJ, Zuurmond WWA, van der Heide A, Perez RSGM, Rietjens JAC. Pressure during decision making of continuous sedation in end-of-life situations in Dutch general practice. BMC Family Practice. 2012;13:68-74. DOI: 10.1186/1471-2296-13-68

[12] Cherny N. Sedation in response to refractory existential distress: Walking the fine line. Journal of Pain and Symptom Management. Commentary. 1998;16(6):404-406. DOI: http://dx.doi.org/10.1016/S0885-3924(98)00114-6

[13] Morita T, Akeki T, Sugawara Y, Chihara S, Uchitomi Y. Practice and attitude of Japanese oncologists and palliative care physicians concerning terminal sedation: A nationwide survey. Journal of Clinical Oncology. 2002;20:758-764. DOI: 10.1200/JCO.2002.20.3.758

[14] Ogden TH, editor. L'identificazione proiettiva e la tecnica psicoterapeutica. Italian translation by Maraini, D. [Projective Identification and Psychotherapeutic Technique. Northvale N.J.: Jason Aronson Inc. Publisher; 1991]. Roma: Astrolabio; 1994. pp. 1-199

[15] Bion WR, editors. Learning from Experience. Karnac Books Ltd; London. 1984. p. 111

[16] Grinberg L. Countertransference and projective counteridentification. Contemporary Psychoanalysis. 1979;15(2):226-247

[17] Searles H, editors. Countertransference and Related Subject: Selected Papers. New York: International Universities Press; 1979. p. 625

[18] Dosamantes I. The intersubjective relationship between therapist and patient: A key to understanding denied and denigrated aspects of the patient's self. The Arts in Psychotherapy. 1992;19:359-365. https://doi.org/10.1016/0197-4556(92)90031-I

[19] Charon R. Narrative medicine. A model for empathy, reflection, profession and trust. Journal of American Medical Association. 2001;17:1897-1902. DOI: 10.1001/jama.286.15.1897

[20] Ferro A, Vender S, editors. La terra di nessuno fra psichiatria e psicoterapia [No man'sland Between Psychiatric and Psychotherapy]. Torino: Bollati Boringhieri; 2010. p. 249

[21] Pruzinsky T, Cash TF. Understanding body images: Historical and contemporary perspectives. In: Cash TF, Pruzinsky T, editors. Body Images: A Handbook of Theory, Research and Clinical Practice. New York: Guilford Press; 2002. pp. 3-12

[22] Arnold EM, Artin KA, Persona JL, Griffith DL. Consideration of hastening death among hospice patients and their families. Journal of Pain and Symptom Management. 2004;6:523-532. DOI: 10.1016/j.jpainsymman.2003.10.010

[23] O'Mahoni S, Goulet J, Kornblith A, Abbatiello G, Clarke B, Kless-Siegel S, Breibart W, Payne R. Desire for hastened death, cancer pain and depression: Report of a longitudinal observational study. Journal of Pain and Symptom Management. 2005;29(5):446-457. DOI: 10.1016/j.jpainsymman.2004.08.010

[24] Rodin G, Lo C, Mikulincer M, Donner A, Gagliese L, Zimmermann C. Pathways to distress: The multiple determinants of depression, hopelessness and the desire for hastened death in metastatic cancer patients. Social Science & Medicine. 2009;68:562-569. DOI: 10.1016/j.socscimed.2008.10.037

[25] Ohnsorge K, Gudat H, Rehmenn-Sutter C. Intention in wishes to die: Analysis and typology. A report of 30 qualitative case studies of terminally ill cancer patients in palliative care. Psycho-Oncology. 2014;23:1021-1026. DOI: 10.1002/pon.3524

[26] Ohnsorge K, Gudat H, Rehmenn-Sutter C. What a wish to die can mean: Reasons, meanings and functions of wishes to die, reported form 30 qualitative case studies of terminally ill cancer patients in palliative care. BMC Palliative Care. 2014;13:38-52. DOI: 10.1186/1472-684X-13-38

[27] Proske U, Gandevia SC. The proprioceptive senses: Their roles in signaling body shape, body position and movement, and muscle force. Physiological Review. 2012;92:1651-1697. DOI: 10.1152/physrev.00048.2011

[28] van Lommel PI. Near death experience, consciousness and the brain. A new concept about continuity of our consciousness based on recent scientific research on NDE in survivors of cardiac arrest. World Futures. 2006;62:134-151. DOI: 10.1080/02604020500412808. Available from: http://www.deanradin.com/evidence/vanLommel2006.pdf [Accessed: April 2017]

[29] Scholz J, Woolf CJ. The neuropathic pain triad: Neurons, immune cells and glia. Nature Neuroscience. 2007;10:1361-1368. DOI: 10.1038/nn1992

[30] Kullmann DM, Moreau AW, Bakiri Y, Nicholson E. Plasticity of inhibition. Neuron. 2012;75:951-962. DOI: 10.1016/j.neuron.2012.07.030

[31] Sabato AF, editors. Dolore basi molecolari [Pain and Molecular basis]. Roma: CIC Edizioni Internazionali; 2010. p. 372

[32] Greyson B. Dissociation in people who have near-death experience: Out of their bodies or out of their minds? Lancet. 2000;355:460-463. DOI: 10.1016/S0140-6736(00)82013-9

[33] Blanke O, Landis T, Spinelli L, Seeck M. Out-of-body experience and autoscopy of neurological origin. Brain. 2004;127:243-258. DOI: 10.1093/brain/awh040

[34] Pollak T. The "body-container": A new perspective on the "body-ego". International Journal of Psychoanalysis. 2009;90(3):487-506. DOI: 10.1111/j.1745-8315.2009.00129.x

[35] Endrizzi C, Ghelleri V, Palella M, D'Amico G. Movement psychotherapy in a hospice: Two case studies. Body, Movement and Dance in Psychotherapy. 2016;11(1):46-59. http://dx.doi.org/10.1080/17432979.2015.1110534

[36] Endrizzi C, Senore C, D'Amico G, Palella M. Factors associated with decision-making process in palliative sedation therapy. The experience of an Italian hospice struggling with balancing various individual autonomies. Cogent Medicine. 2017;4(1290307):1-15. DOI: 2331205X.2017.1290307

[37] Surbone A. Truth telling to the patient. Journal of American Medical Association JAMA. 1992;268:1661-1662. DOI: 10.1001/jama.1992.03490130049015

[38] Nunez-Olarte JN, JGuillén DG. Cultural issues and ethical dilemmas in palliative and end-of-life care in Spain. Cancer Control. 2001;8:46-54

[39] Grassi L, Giraldi T, Messina EG, Magnani K, Valle E, Cartei G. Physicians' attitudes to and problem with truth-telling to cancer patients. Supportive Care Cancer. 2000;8:40-45. DOI: 10.1007/s005209900067

[40] Cherny N, Catane R. Attitudes of medical oncologists toward palliative care for patients with advanced and incurable cancer. Cancer. 2003;98(11):2502-2510. DOI: 10.1002/cncr.11815

[41] Asai M, Morita T, Akechi T, Sugawara Y, Fujimori M, Akizuki N, et al. Burnout and psychiatric morbidity among physicians engaged in end-of-life for cancer patients: A cross-sectional nationwide survey in Japan. Psycho-Oncology. 2007;16:421-428. DOI: 10.1002/pon.1066

[42] Endrizzi C, Ghelleri V, Palella M, Cossino P, D'Amico G. Health workers faced with death: The influence of training on the language employed in the passage from life to death. Body, Movement and Dance in Psychotherapy. 2014;9(2):74-81. http://dx.doi.org/10.1080/17432979.2014.897999

Chapter 2

# Ethics in Palliative Care

Padmashri Rastogi

Additional information is available at the end of the chapter

http://dx.doi.org/10.5772/intechopen.70508

*"Should you shield the canyons from the windstorm, you would never see the true beauty of their carving".*
*Elizabeth Kubler Ross*

**Abstract**

In 1959, Victor Frankl considered universal facts of life to be suffering, death and existential guilt and called it the "tragic triad". Life is suffering, as Lord Buddha concluded. Palliative care tries to reduce this suffering which increases even more near the end of life. Severe pain can compromise the quality of life. Ethicist will guard against counter phobic determination to treat pain as health care team undertreats the pain are worried about excessive sedation and concern for hastening death. Palliative care is best for controlling the symptoms in these difficult situations. Even when goals of care are so clear, still there are lots of ethical question. Most common reasons are conflicts in values between physician and patient or patient and his family. There can also be conflict in expectations. Here we have described ethical issues with ethical analysis with few common clinical scenarios to help the reader associate these in their practice.

**Keywords:** good death, suffering, Ulysses contract, dementia, do not attempt resuscitation (DNAR), double effect, metaphysician

## 1. Introduction

Medical ethics is a scholarly inquiry regarding which moral values and specific ethical principles will apply in each situation. In palliative care, the goal should be to let the patient maintain their dignity and hope while they are here alive. Afterwards, when the time comes, death should be peaceful, pain-free and without any suffering. If the patient can be surrounded by his loved ones and had time to say Good byes, it is fortunate. Most people will call this a "Good Death".

The duration of symptom management is a very important factor in patient care. Ideally, with an increase in life-span, the expectation would be a prolonged healthy life followed by a short period of illness and quick death. Along with an increase in healthy phase, the period of the chronic disease is significantly prolonged, followed by slower death. Palliative care is offered to those whose suffering can be relieved by special care while they continue with active treatment of their disease. Palliative care does not require a life expectancy of <6 months. Hospice provides only comfort care when life expectancy is around 6 months. It all started in the 1940s, when Cecily Saunders recognized the need for a place where terminally ill patients can be cared for while maintaining their dignity, functional status, and moral uplift by living well till the time comes. In 1967, after she became a physician, she opened St Christopher Hospice [1]. In 1965, Elisabeth Kubler Ross joined the University of Chicago. In 1969 she published her book "On Death and Dying". Her passion for her work on terminally ill patients, dying, and death took her on the roller coaster ride of her career where she published many books on the topic. She wrote her first book on the mysteries of life and living in 2000 [2]. Attention to the process of dying was pioneered by Dame Saunders and Dr Ross.

## 2. Ethical issues in palliative care

Usually, most of the ethical inquiries of the day are resolved without going into any principle or theory of ethics. Life will be sacred for some at all cost. Others seek happiness. It is the patient's right to decide for themselves. Other persons may have value to believe the right action is the one which will bring maximum happiness for the most number of people. The sanctity of life makes it our duty to preserve and prolong life, but it cannot be absolute. Rather, it must depend on the situation. If only life preservation will remain the goal, then the suffering at the end of life will be prolonged as well. In another way, some conditions will prolong the process of dying. The principle of utility, when used, will promote happiness in as many persons as possible. It does not include health care provider's own happiness. There can be two kinds of utilitarianism in which action is judged by the principle of utility. Rule utilitarianism applies the principle of utility through a set of rules which will bring maximum overall happiness [3].

### 2.1. Autonomy for choice of living arrangement

After being in palliative care for a short duration, it was proposed that Mr R L move to a nursing home for continuation of pain medication and getting help in activities of daily living. He refused to go to the nursing home and requested to be discharged home. He asked his wife if she was okay with his decision of not to go to the nursing home and assured her that he would no longer be a burden to her with getting help from the home health services. That night Mr R. L. took all his pills for pain, insomnia, and anxiety along with a bottle of Tylenol. In the morning, his wife found him in deep sleep in his bed, tucked in the blanket, bible on the side table. She removed the blanket to wake him up and saw him dressed in a white shirt and black suit with socks and shoes, like he was going to church. At that moment, she realized that he has gone, indeed.

Ethical issues in this case are:

- Should a patient have control over timing of death when it is imminent anyways?
- Should we respect their choice?
- Should he go to the nursing home, which would have made everyone happy other than him?

On a cursory view, it appears that medical system failed him. Once we analyze it ethically, the patient's wishes have been respected following the principles of autonomy and dignity. Principle of justice is evident when he was treated like anyone else with care and compassion. Doctor and nurses gave their advice for him to go to the nursing home but when patient expressed that he would prefer to go home, they did not force him to go to the nursing home. It does not mean that patient will be safe or his decision is the alternative I would suggest but it is where ethics has a crucial role. This exemplifies utilitarianism as he did not spend his savings on a nursing home, making his wife happy. Since he did not have to go to a nursing home, he was happy as well. If he decided to end his life in the isolation of his room without any involvement of others, it was his choice. He did not apparently suffer and as per discussion with his wife, this was a good death for him [4].

The principle of justice proposes equal treatment and care for all those in the similar situation. The goal of palliative care is to relieve suffering. Suffering is a reaction to something which causes pain: physical, mental, emotional, or moral. The reaction depends on the person. The principle of justice demands the similar treatment of persons of similar conditions, but the ethics of palliative care permits discretion on the part of the physician, as treatment is tailored to the patient. St Augustine has described it beautifully in City of God.

> *"… though exposed to the same anguish, virtue and vice are not the same thing. For as the same fire causes gold to glow brightly, and chaff to smoke; and under the same flail the straw is beaten small, while the grain is cleansed… So material a difference does it make, not what ills are suffered, but what kind of man suffers them. For, stirred up with the same movement, mud exhales a horrible stench, and ointment emits a fragrant odor".*

Suffering in the same person can be perceived differently and cause significant challenges in management. In the following scenario, would you agree that the patient is suffering or is the longevity worth this suffering?

### 2.2. Silent suffering in dementia?

Mr JA had a stroke at the age of 54. For the last 11 years, having lived in a nursing facility, he has suffered more strokes and had advanced vascular dementia for last 4 years. He stopped eating, and, when fed, he would open his mouth but neither chewed nor swallowed. At that time, a discussion was held regarding artificial nutrition and hydration. The patient's Medical Power of Attorney (MPOA), his daughter, insisted on it and was not willing to consider anything further. Having a Gastric (G) tube connected to the nutrition bottle, JA could no longer control his activities as feeding had to be planned around by the nurses' schedule. In the last 4 months, he had pulled out his G tube 11 times, leaving him without food or water for hours until it could be replaced. To prevent dehydration, he requires Intravenous (IV) fluids during these times. When a nurse comes to place the IV line, he makes it apparent that he does not want the IV placed. To prevent him from pulling the IV line, he is physically constrained by hand restraints.

The medical staff caring for him believed that the patient was suffering. He was not happy with the tube in his stomach, frequent intravenous needle placement, or his hands restraints. His daughter, who came on the weekends to see him, found him completely comfortable and saw no issues with the procedures being done. She always brought chocolate for him, which he enjoyed, and he was always happy to see her.

The ethical concerns would be:

- Was the patient suffering?
- Since he has dementia and may not be capable of informed consent, should the health care team follow his daughter's instructions?

At times, doing nothing is the best discourse, but very difficult in practice. Placing the feeding tube in this case is controversial as it can be a source of suffering, but has been necessary in sustaining the patient's life. Now, the patient can decide about their quality of life and depending on the answer, whether sustaining his life is beneficial [5].

Deciding when to give all options, regardless of benefit, and when not to offer all options is dependent on the analysis of a patient's values, living will, and the benefit/risk ratio. It also depends on whether a surrogate/health care agent is making substitutive judgment or if his/her judgment is according to selfish motives. Jay Katz mentions a case where even useful options were not presented.

"Immediately prior to our meeting, the nephrologist had examined a French peasant who lived some 40 miles outside of Paris and suffered from chronic renal failure. The condition was a rapidly progressive one and would soon lead to death if not placed on dialysis. Yet the patient was not offered this option. Instead, he was told that no medical treatment existed that would help him. When I asked the nephrologist, he reacted with surprise, like the answer was self-evident: 'To say more would have been cruel. Peasants do not adjust well to a permanent move to a large city'" [6].

Ethically speaking, to make a choice for the patient is paternalism, but the physician may justify it as his fiduciary duty to not cause mental suffering. To see the same action by various angles makes it clearer. It is possible that in a few cases, that the "doctor knows best" indeed. The autonomy of the patient will not be respected for the sake of beneficence. At many times, the treatment of a disease causes more suffering than the disease itself.

### 2.3. Iatrogenic pain

89-year-old JL, a man with a pressure ulcer on his sacral area and both heels require dressing at least once a day. He cries with pain whenever he is turned for dressing changes. It appears that the dressing hurts him as he can be turned other times without any outcry. The patient's life expectancy is limited as his albumin has dropped to 1.2, hemoglobin 8, and total cholesterol 92. Nursing staff feel that the patient is in pain when they do his dressings and want to

http://dx.doi.org/10.5772/intechopen.70508

decrease the frequency of dressing. But the doctor is concerned about sepsis if he is not provided with the standard of care.

An ethics consultant or palliative care physician can conduct an interdisciplinary meeting and discuss goals of care as well as safe and judicious use of pain medications that is enough to control pain.

When a medication is given for one effect which is needed by the patient, but the dosage that is needed to produce that therapeutic effect can cause other serious effects, that is, suppression of breathing or even death, it is known as "double effect". Intention is important for the double effect to apply.

Resuscitation may not be medically indicated even though patient and MPOA have not given permission for "Do not resuscitate" orders.

### 2.4. Simply dead

84-year old Mrs ND had been in palliative care for 11 days with aphasia, dysphagia, and inability to turn. Otherwise, she could move in bed although too weak to stand. Physical therapy transferred her to a wheelchair where she could sit for several hours every day. She had a gastric tube, Foley catheter, and inhaled oxygen. Apparently, she suffered from hypoxic brain injury. Since she did not communication in any way, it was hard to assess her decision making capacity. Her daughter, the MPOA refused to make her Do Not Attempt Resuscitation (DNAR) as she believed that her mother will recover from this episode. This morning Mrs ND was found to be breathing rapidly with fever of 104°F on morning rounds by the nursing staff. They called 911 and transferred her to the nearest hospital. However, as she was being transported she stopped breathing. As they had already reached the emergency department, she was handed over to the ED physician who called for the code cart. She was pale and pulseless without a heartbeat and not breathing, and the pupils of both eyes were dilated and fixed. She had a fever of 104° last night prior to transfer. It appeared that she had died on the way to the hospital during transfer. What should the physician do?

Choices for the physician:

**a.** Declare her dead

**b.** She is full code, so he should try resuscitation.

**c.** As she is full code, she should be intubated even if there is no response.

Mrs ND could have been in a skilled nursing home and receive extensive physical therapy, but her daughter wants to keep her comfortable while getting physical therapy, allowing only as much as Mrs ND could tolerate comfortably.

Though, legally, she has the right to resuscitation unless the physician is sure of futility. In this case, calling code is okay. CPR and, if qualified, defibrillation is acceptable, but if there is no response, then intubation will not be necessary. The physician fulfills the patient's and daughter's goal of care to keep Mrs ND comfortable by granting her a peaceful death. He did not accelerate or hasten death, but when the situation presented itself and there were no chances of recovery, there was no use of intubation or pacemaker. The physician called the chaplain and her daughter. The daughter was appreciative that the physician attended to her mother promptly and did what was best for her mother. This was a difficult decision to make, but the physician knew that the patient had all the signs of death and, given her previous brain damage, she would not tolerate this anoxia for so many minutes. Hence, he let her go peacefully. Sometimes when middle ground is chosen between paternalism and autonomy, it is known as "mutual autonomy". [7]

### 2.5. Ethics of dementia in palliative care

Dementia is one diagnosis that looks just right for palliative care. There are no goals left in life except to live happily till the end. Agitation or frustration can be an occasional problem when a person cannot express themselves. Many patients with dementia qualify for hospice and palliative care and in fact, improve in this nurturing environment. Sadly, only 20% of referrals to hospice/palliative care is for non-cancer patients [8]. On average, stay of patients with dementia is shorter than their cancer counterpart. Dementia is not recognized as terminal illness as the patient does not go to the doctor, patient is unaware of the problem Caretakers maintain their hygiene and keep them well fed, not an easy task.

> I want to tell you how much
>
> I miss my mother.
>
> Bits of her are still there.
>
> I miss her most when
>
> I am sitting across from her.
>
> Candy Crawley

In modern facilities, there are various activities for these patients. When person starts withdrawing from social activities, one should suspect depression or increasing neurocognitive deficits [9]. Ethics is vital for managing these patients as it is common to have a controversy over what is best for the patient.

> Time, you enjoy wasting is not a wasted time.
> Marth Troly-Curtin, Phrynette Married

Mr V was transported to geriatric nursing home as he was increasingly isolated, inactive, stayed bed-ridden, avoiding eye contact, and hardly speaking. Physical therapy tried the Merry Walker on him, and he suddenly realized that he could move on his own, making him very happy. He needed supervision while using the Merry Walker, hence he could only use it for 30–60 minutes per day. When the social worker and nurse noticed the change in Mr V's personality, they discussed the matter with visiting family members. Consequently, his family requested that he should be permitted to use the Merry Walker for a longer duration. The concern of restraints did not bother Mr V or his family, as he feels safe in the cloth restraint which goes across his chest. Increased risk of fall while using the Merry Walker is a concern, but, as the patient is already at high fall risk, it is uncertain that the Merry Walker increases this risk. This cloth restraint is strong and cues the patient to only move forward facing. Since the family is willing to assume both the risks, is it ethical to put advanced dementia patient in a Merry Walker with group supervision and can family be permitted to assume these responsibilities?

When the clinician accepts either the patient's or health-care proxy's decision, it shows respect for the patient and the doctrine of self-determination for which Justice Cardozo wrote: "Every human being of adult years and sound mind has a right to determine what shall be done with his own body" (1914) [10].

Here, the physician must agree to the same risk that the patient is willing to take although the physician does have the autonomy not to be forced to recommend a device in suboptimal conditions. It is of note that the therapist initiated the use of this device, and it benefitted the patient tremendously. According to ethical analysis, the benefit-risk ratio clearly tilts toward benefit; hence, the Merry Walker may be prescribed under group supervision with the consent from a surrogate to whom risks and disadvantages of the Merry Walker have been described in detail [11].

Here, many people will turn to the Law for a solution. The law appears clear and unambiguous in its answers. On the other hand, Law keeps changing with time and jurisdiction, and it has not defined all our activities as lawful or unlawful. Law can demand morally wrong actions, that is, doctors in Nazi Germany [12]. Regarding this case, at least one law suit has been filed against the Merry Walker.

Ethics consult appear unique until it is broken down into values and principles. As in this example, the ethical question is: can a surrogate consent for risk taken by the patient when he uses the device? This question was answered by court in a case of Karen B Quinlan when his adoptive parents were permitted to withdraw life support based on substitutive decision. As for the clinician's side, a person in palliative care is there for quality of life, and if the Merry Walker makes him energetic and happy without discomfort, prescribing Merry Walker with group supervision should be within the clinician's comfort zone.

While interest in caring for the dying has been increasing in the medical field, avoidance of death and dying is the norm for society in general, resulting in 29% of persons dying in the hospital and the average terminal admissions lasting 7.9 days in 2010 [8]. Focus on prolonging the life became so intense that humane physician Dr Walby had to make way for Dr House on Television.

> "When the world says, 'Give up', Hope whispers, 'Try it one more time'".
>
> Anonymous

### 2.6. Different set of goals

Mr L was transferred from acute care to a long-term care community center with diminished mobility. While in acute care, he was hooked up to intravenous lines and only received passive movement therapy. Active movement physical therapy was started, but the patient was not interested. After 2 weeks of physical therapy, the patient could transfer himself from the bed to wheel chair with minimal assistance. He did not start walking with a walker as he used to do before, but he was happy to move in his manual wheel chair. He showed no interest in physical therapy and was in pain during exercises. He was started on a dose of Tylenol prior to exercise time which helped, but he remained tense during exercises and walking with physical therapist. As he has not achieved his functional goal of walking with a walker, should one continue physical therapy despite his obvious dislike for it?

Palliative care provides comfort care to the patient under the principle of *Primum no nocere*. Non-maleficence is the most important principle out of four guiding principles of ethical decision making. The case of Mr L makes a case of slow improvement. If the physical therapy is continued, as it has been optimized, and the patient is in pain during therapy, there is no reason to continue physical therapy now. The counter argument to this approach is that by providing physical therapy, the outcome and expectations may be different for the provider and the patient. Small improvements in endurance where he can stand on his own by holding the side of the bed for half a minute may mean a lot to him as he can then use a bedside commode. A small step for the provider can be a big difference in quality of life for the patient. This will advocate for the continued physical therapy.

> One thing is certain and the, rest is lies.
>
> Omair

Death appears in many guises. To some, it is a relief from chronic pain and suffering. To others, it may be sudden and unexpected [13]. It could be traumatic and shocking. When activities of daily living can be performed without assistance, one need to be able to get out of bed or chair, use the toilet, bathe, groom, dress, eat, and walk. Most people will lose Independent Activities of Daily Living which are: shop, cook, do laundry for himself, maintain housekeeping, take medications for himself, make phone calls, travel, and handle his finances.

> There are all kinds of futures.
>
> There is a hoped-for future,
>
> there is a feared future,
>
> there is a predictable future,
>
> and there is an unimagined future.
>
> - Werner Erhard

### 2.7. Ethics of Ulysses' contract

Mr S is 63-year-old lawyer who had been very successful in his personal life and career. He had been living with amyotrophic lateral sclerosis (ALS) for last 3 years. Three years ago, he could still walk though awkwardly, both his arms dangled with no strength. He realized that accelerated pace of ALS is going to be devastating. On his next visit to the doctor, he requested no resuscitation and no life support or sustaining treatment in any circumstances. He wanted to be sure that he would never be on respirator. His doctor suggested Ulysses contract so even if he would like to change his decision about life support, only his current wishes would be honored. S asked his doctor to help him take his life. His doctor explains the law and offered him palliative care through inpatient hospice. Even though he is not eligible in conventional sense for hospice, his doctor helps him with the admission so that he can achieve a good death prior to intense suffering and saves him from committing suicide.

Ulysses also known as Odysseus is famous for his brilliant plan of escaping from the Sirens. Songs of the Sirens were beyond humans resolve to stay away and that's how always resulted in shipwreck at the sharp rocky island of Sirens. To save himself Ulysses asked his men to tie him to the ships mast and put wax in all the sailors' ears so that they could row but not hear. Ulysses contract is used to ensure implementation of previously carefully thought plan and not get influenced by the future weaknesses. There are many ethical questions and it should not be used widely [14].

Mr S was feeling increasing isolation, loss of interest of his treating team, and had lost all hope. He was requiring more assistance from his wife, she did it cheerfully without complaining. When they discussed what was coming, she remained optimistic. For the patient's good, he was referred early than normally indicated due to this unique situation of knowing the progression of disease. Hence, he feels lonely even when surrounded by his friends and family. The physician facilitates the transition for patient to achieve his goals.

Basic knowledge of ethics should be the requirement for all clinicians, more so for people working in an Emergency Department (ED). Though there are lots of venues to get into urgent decision making for life and death, there is nothing like a patient brought by ambulance, alone who is in respiratory failure. Patients on palliative care usually do not end up at the emergency department. On rare occasions, a doctor may ask a patient to go to ED as a terminally ill patient reflects their defeat to maintain health and by having no magic bullet to fix things, causes avoidance of the patient. Knowing the duration of suffering brings desire to do more in the physicians like in child birth, traumatic injury or post-operative pain [15].

> Choose your future and take action. Be the hammer, not the nail
>
> - Jonathan Lockwood Hui

### 2.8. Validity of advance directives

Mr P was brought to the emergency department by ambulance. He was 87-year-old, comes with pneumonia and end stage chronic obstructive pulmonary disease. There was a Do not intubate order, had not been touched in last 10 years. Patient was not receiving care here in last 10 years. Patient had been brought alone and patient was responding only to pain. His son, his health care agent arrived shortly. Patient was under palliative care, he had progressively worsened and was now in respiratory distress. The physician offered intubation, the patient was unable to speak and his health care agent asks for comfort care. What should the physician do?

Ethical dilemma arises when patient's autonomous decision is causing him harm. In this scenario, it may cost his life. If he had refused the use of invasive device, he should not get one. Doctors are trained to try to conquer death so it is hard on him to not intubate and save him. Physician has a decade old written directive from patient. Ethical question is, whether it is ever justifiable to overrule a patient's refusal for his own good? [16]. Son agrees with his father's wishes. Principles involved here are: Patient's self-determination, patients' bill of rights, physician's duty to do good and first do not harm. Even if physician intubated him, chances of meaningful recovery were very less. Then physician also violates patient's request as well as decision of his health care agent. If recently he changed his mind and wanted intubation, then Mr P did not get that chance. End of life issues can be complicated. Physicians are discouraged to make unilateral decisions even in complex situations or when they have irreconcilable differences with patient and/or surrogate.

Good-life till the end is good death. Death is individual. A person may just want his bed and his dog at the time of death. Another person may want to be at the beach. Yet another person may wish for a day without any pain on the day of death.

> Also, I would like a doctor who is not only talented physician, but a bit of metaphysician too. Someone who can treat body and soul.
>
> Anatole Broyard

### 2.9. Autonomy vs beneficence

A 47-year-old male patient requests to go home without ventilator. He has been ventilator dependent for many years. He has paralysis below T10. Now, he has decided that he does not see any benefit in prolonging life when all he can move is his upper body. Nurses tried to tell him that he will get anxious without any medication in hand, Patient was asking to do withdrawal of life support as he is reaching home, so he can die peacefully at home without any tubes. It was decided that a hospice nurse will go along with the patient and give medication according to his needs, she will be in contact with his doctor all this time. Bioethics is in agreement with achieving the patient's goals.

Pain control remains a challenge even for palliative care. It is commonly noticed that patients require higher opioid dose than their usual dose. It is ethical to give enough pain medication to control the pain while keeping an eye for a placement making sure that intravenous line is indeed in vein and not blocked so that the dosage increase should increase the effectiveness of pain medication. Dyspnea or air hunger should be treated with anxiolytic or morphine. Again, the dosage required may be way higher on occasions, so far it is documented clearly about symptoms, and what is the goal, there is no ceiling for the dosage. If intention is to control pain and dyspnea, increased dosage of these medications may diminish respiratory drive to the point of death, this is known as double effect, not physician-assisted death.

> *"We want autonomy for ourselves and safety for those we love. That remains the main problem and paradox for the frail. Many of the things that we want for those we care about are the things that we would oppose for ourselves because they would infringe upon our sense of self"* [17].

### 2.10. Vegetative state and choice of surrogate decision maker

Mrs NC was an elegant mother of four, now living alone at the house since her children had moved out and her husband had died in line of duty 15 years ago working in armed forces. One day, while speaking to her daughter, she suddenly started having gurgling noises and the phone fell from her hand. Her daughter called 911 and went to emergency department. Mrs NC was breathing on her own, eyes closed, no deformity of face, laying on her back. A quick physical by the emergency physician elicited no response to cortical functions, her brain stem reflexes were present. After magnetic resonance imaging (MRI), Electroencephalogram (EEG) and vascular studies over next week by the neurologist, she was found to be in vegetative state. She had no advance directive. Having no treatment to reverse damage, palliative care was consulted. Palliative care physician arranged a multidisciplinary meeting that evening. Three children could come. They discussed the goal of care, and it was agreed that Mrs NC did not believe in life support when there are no chances of recovery. She would receive comfort care and no artificial food and water. Her eldest son who came back from his trip was shocked to see his mother just waiting to die, he demanded that everything should be done for her including gastric tube for feeding and to move her out of hospice. What should palliative care do?

If patient does not have decision making capacity the surrogate decision maker should be selected from this list in order of priority:

Health care agent or Medical power of attorney

Court appointed Guardian

Spouse

Adult Children

Parents

Adult siblings

Next close relative or friend

Minor variations can be there according to jurisdiction

Her daughter Nancy lives a block away, while her daughter Julia lives across the town but stays with her mother on weekends. Her son John lives a few miles away but he takes her for groceries, appointments, shopping, and takes her out for dinner. Her eldest son Dennis was traveling for his work at the time of his mother's admission. What should be the order of the preference? Eldest to youngest, boys first then girls or the one who does the most for their mother? The ethical answer is none of the above. All adult children have equal weightage. In the case like this when there is difference of opinion, a family meeting should be called and the question posed is what your mother would decide if she could for herself? Everyone agreed that she would not want to live like this. No change was made and the patient passed away in her sleep by the time meeting was over [10].

Most palliative care physicians handle the stress well. Occasionally, a patient comes along who requires lot more care but his suffering continues. In these cases, a physician maintains their integrity and silently continues to suffer. Moral distress is defined as "the pain or anguish effecting the mind, body or relationships in response to a situation in which the person is aware of a moral problem, acknowledges moral responsibility and makes a moral judgment about the correct action, yet as a result of real or perceived constraints, participates in perceived moral wrongdoing" [18]. Biomedical ethics protects palliative care physicians from significant moral dilemmas but adds some as well.

Clinical Scenario:

> "Student must learn that there are areas of experience where we know that uncertainty is the certainty".
>
> James B Conant [6]

Providing care to those with rare diseases which are devastating to the person and family yet do not follow typical path of morbidity and mortality. Typical markers of impending death do not appear until very late.

Under the care of Doctor Mims, Ms. SM had stayed in a mental health lock down facility for 5 weeks. **The doctor** was pleased with the control of her volatile mood, depression, and anxiety, but now calm she is focused on leaving this controlled area. Hence a palliative care consult was placed for inpatient care but was not approved. Ms SM was diagnosed with Huntington's Chorea for the last 4 years. She was doing well until last year when she started to exhibit unpredictable, unprovoked burst of aggressive behavior, limiting her choices for living. She needed strong antipsychotics to calm her down. She started to lose her balance and needed help in ADLs. Her appetite remained good and she did not lose weight. She was not meeting the criteria for palliative care and hospice. In general, indicators for imminent death are weight loss, pressure ulcers, signs of nutritional deficiency, anemia and/or uremia, which are not present in Ms. SM.

Here the issue is that this patient will benefit from comfort care early on to save suffering from the now predictable down spiral course of the disease. Huntington's Chorea is a rapidly progressive neurodegenerative disease with autosomal dominant transmission. Bioethics is used for justice by ensuring palliative care to the individuals according to their need. A strict policy criterion does not work in all institutions or for all patients. The patient values were to maintain her dignity and independence and did not want life support if her disease advances. Concerned about the disease and with the 50% possibility of transmitting to the next generation, she did not marry and had no children. She had worked full-time in her adult life and had left her assets with her mother, showing the good relationship between the two. The criteria for palliative care in Huntington's Chorea are a little different. A patient qualifies for palliative and hospice care when they start to require:

Assistance for ambulation and other activities of daily living ADLs, like dressing

Loss of control over urination and defecation

Difficulty in communication

Despite having dementia, a person with Huntington's disease usually recognizes a familiar song, prayer, church, and minister of long duration. The focus should be at quality of life at the end stage of the disease. After a short delay, the patient was admitted to palliative care, where she stayed until her death.

Cure few, treats most, and comfort always. The goal of medicine is healing of sick. Healing includes cure of physical inflictions along with psychosocial and/or spiritual needs. The cure

Huntington's disease is an autosomal dominant disease transmitted by one of the parents. Problem has been mapped to short arm of chromosome 4, where sequence of Cytosine-Adenosine-Guanine (CAG) is repeated. Normally CAG is repeated 11–34 times, median being 19. When it is repeated 35–39, it is diagnostic of Huntington's Disease. Severity of the disease proportionately increases with the number of repeat sequence [19].

of ailment is ideal. When a cure is not possible, the physician continues to treat to minimize the impact of disease. When death is imminent, the physician comes by to assure his presence, reassure peaceful transition, to acknowledge patient's relevance in life and emphasizing his company till the end. Before the advent of clinical ethics and the expansion of bioethics, death was not talked about, as it would not happen if not mentioned [20]. Now and for the last 40 years, the patient gets to choose the type of care he wants at the end of life. The patient gets to decide which life sustaining treatment he will like if needed. Now, the presumption is that the patient understands the condition and options well enough to decide on his own [21]. Most of the patients would ask their clinicians for advice. The therapeutic relation between doctor and patient is unique and physician has a fiduciary duty to safeguard interests of his patients.

In conclusion, ethics is an integral part of end of life care, same as palliative care and hospice. Ethical scenario described above only cover few issues. One important ethical topic in palliative care is difference between withholding and withdrawal of care. Though they seem similar, in practice, it is easy not to start life support as opposed to withdrawal. Philosopher Dan Brock gives a very nice example. A man is being taken in ambulance and in one version wife reaches the Emergency department at the same time as her husband and shows do not attempt resuscitation (DNAR) order, physician provides comfort care only. In second version, wife gets caught in traffic and gets late to emergency room, her husband is intubated at the time, she shows the same DNAR order and physician refuses to extubate him to let him die. As Brock explains: do not the very same circumstances that justified not placing the patient on ventilator now justify taking him off of it?

In writer's view, if doctor and patient will have long-term relationship, same doctor will manage inpatient and outpatient, the relationship will solve most of the problems of end of life care. Problems arise when patient has no faith in the doctor and doctor does not have a clue about patient's values. Both of these need time to develop, and time is one thing dying patient does not have.

Note the view expressed in this chapter do not represent those of US federal government or the Department of Veteran Affairs and are purely my own personal views. All cases are fictionalized, although inspired by a combination of real cases seen in clinical practice by myself or others.

## Author details

Padmashri Rastogi[1,2*]

*Address all correspondence to: 123123qr@gmail.com

1 North Texas Health Care System, Dallas, USA

2 Department of Internal Medicine, UT Southwestern Medical Centre, Dallas, USA

## References

[1] Drought TS, Koenig BA. "Choice" in end-of-life decision making: Researching fact or fiction? Gerontologist. 2002;**42**(Spec No 3):114-128

[2] [Internet]. 2016. Available from: https://www.nhpco.org/history-hospice-care [Accessed: 2017-07-07] History of Hospice Care, National Hospice and Palliative Care Association, 3-28-2016

[3] Sugarman J, Sulmasy DP. Methods in Medical Ethics. 2nd ed. Washington, DC: Georgetown University Press; 2010;112-117

[4] Benjamin M, Curtis J. Ethics in Nursing: Cases, Principles, and Reasoning. New York: Oxford University Press, Inc.; 2010

[5] Gunderman RB. Is suffering the enemy? Hastings Center Report. 2002;**32**:40-44. DOI: 10.2307/3528523

[6] Jay Katz J. The Silent World of Doctor and Patient. Baltimore: Johns Hopkins University Press; 2002. p. 186

[7] Pellegrino ED, Thomasma DC. For the Patient's Good: The Restoration of Beneficence in Health Care. New York, Oxford University Press 1988;142-147

[8] Tang VL, French CJ, Cipher DJ, Rastogi P. Trends in hospice referral and length of stay at a veterans hospital over the past decade. The American Journal of Hospice & Palliative Care. 2013;**30**(5):432-436. DOI: 10.1177/1049909112453642

[9] Congedo M, Causarano RI, Alberti F, et al. Ethical issues in end of life treatments for patients with dementia. European Journal of Neurology. 2010;**17**(6):774-779. DOI: 10.1111/j.1468-1331.2010.02991.x

[10] Faden RR, Beauchamp T. A History and Theory of Informed Consent. Oxford: Oxford University Press; 1989. p. 123

[11] A Different Take on Walkers—Alzheimer's and Dementia [Internet]. 2011. Available from: http://www.alzheimersreadingroom.com/2011/04/different-take-on-walkers.html [Accessed: 2017-07-07]

[12] Kantor JE. Medical Ethics for Physicians-in-Training. New York City: Springer; 1989. pp. 1-6

[13] Christiaan Bernard C. Good Life Good Death: A Doctor's Case for Euthanasia and Suicide. Englewood Cliffs: Prentice Hall Trade; 1980

[14] Ulysses Contract Mindfulness Map I Putting Wisdom to Work book [Internet]. Available from: http://policypillars.com/self-help-tools/13-pillar-power-personal-growth-worksheet.html [Accessed: 2017-07-07]

[15] Novack DH, Plumer R, Smith RL, Ochitill H, Morrow GR, Bennett JM. Changes in physicians' attitudes toward telling the cancer patient. JAMA. 1979;**241**(9):897-900

[16] Dewolf Bosek MS. When respecting patient autonomy may not be in the patient's best interest. JONA'S Healthcare Law, Ethics and Regulation. 2007;**9**(2):46-49. DOI: 10.1097/01.NHL.0000277199.78814.fb

[17] Gawande A. Being Mortal. Metropolitan Books, Henry Holt and Company, New York. 2014;p. 106

[18] Rushton CH, Kaszniak AW, Halifax JS. A framework for understanding moral distress among palliative care clinicians. Journal of Palliative Medicine. 2013;**16**(9):1074-1079. DOI: 10.1089/jpm.2012.0490

[19] Ropper A, Samuels M, Klein J. Adams and Victor's Principles of Neurology. 10th ed. New York City: McGraw-Hill Education/Medical; 2014. p. 1076

[20] Blinderman CD, Billings JA. Comfort care for patients dying in the hospital. The New England Journal of Medicine. 2015;**373**(26):2549-2561. DOI: 10.1056/NEJMra1411746

[21] Quill TE, Miller FG. Palliative Care and Ethics. USA: Oxford University Press; 2014. Difficult decisions near the very end of life, Truog Robert. pp. 188-189

Chapter 3

# Balance Sheets of Suffering in End-of-Life Care

Ger Wackers

Additional information is available at the end of the chapter

http://dx.doi.org/10.5772/intechopen.70222

**Abstract**

Drawing on recent work in cognitive linguistics and social studies of knowledge practices, this chapter explores the various ways in which the figure of a *balance sheet* frames arguments and positions in end-of-life care. Across arguments and positions, there are substantial differences in the kinds of matter that are balanced against each other and the values attributed to them, and which items are allowed as entries on the balance sheet and which are not. A common currency on the balance sheets is human suffering. Comparing Norwegian and Dutch end-of-life care practices, the argument is elaborated by looking at (a) the personal balance sheets of cancer patients, (b) the balance sheets of euthanasia, assisted suicide, and palliative sedation, and (c) the balance sheets that set patient's right to self-determination up against health professional's right to conscience. Finally, the different ways in which the balance sheets are operated are considered with regard to their impact on the level of constraints that the different end-of-life care policies put on patients and health professionals, and how these shape the material conditions of our dying.

**Keywords:** balance sheets of suffering, conceptual blending, modes of ordering, end-of-life care, palliative care, euthanasia, assisted suicide, palliative sedation

## 1. Introduction

Every argument must generate a space in which it can be persuasive, valid, true, or right—a space in which it can be represented. These abstract *spaces of representation* [1] comprise a framing logic, produced data, conceptual structure, and explicit or implicit onto-epistemological and moral positions. They constitute, to use Mark Turner's phrase, comprehensive *hyper-blends* [2], or to use Annemarie Mol and John Law's expression, *modes of ordering* [3]. Several such comprehensive hyper-blends or modes of ordering may exist simultaneously, generating lines of friction, contention, and disagreement [3]. These spaces do not have to be invented *de novo* every time an argument is made. They are available as cultural, narrative, or discursive resources, that is, as collective templates that can be recruited and operated through blending with the particulars of situated arguments at hand.

Drawing on the recent work in cognitive linguistics [2, 4–8] and social studies of knowledge practices [1, 3], in this chapter, the various ways in which the figure of a *balance sheet* and its associated *calculative devices* frames arguments and positions in end-of-life care will be explored. Across arguments and positions, there are substantial differences in the kinds of matter that are balanced against each other and the values attributed to them, and which items are allowed as entries on the balance sheet and which are not.

The arguments about the balance sheets of suffering in end-of-life care that are being developed here are no exception to the requirement that they too need a space in which they can be persuasive, valid, or right. An important feature of "my space" is that it moves away from the long-held assumption that ontology, epistemology, and ethics constitute separate domains, toward a view that takes notions of embodied cognition and the performative nature of discursive-material practices as its point of departure. In the next section, we will make that "move" explicit, before introducing the notions of *conceptual blending* and *modes of ordering*. Following these introductory sections, the figure of the balance sheet as a space in which moral arguments are presented and weighed against each other is introduced. The most common currency on the balance sheets is human suffering. Comparing Norwegian and Dutch end-of-life care practices, the argument elaborates by looking at (a) the personal balance sheets of cancer patients, (b) the balance sheets of euthanasia, assisted suicide, and palliative sedation, and (c) the balance sheets that set patient's right to self-determination up against health professional's right to conscience. Finally, how the different ways in which the balance sheets are operated impact the level of constraints that the different end-of-life care policies put on patients and health professionals, and how they shape the material conditions of our dying are shown.

## 2. From disembodied to embodied cognition and discursive-material practices

We still struggle with the legacy of long-held assumptions about the separateness of question of ontology, epistemology, and ethics. These assumptions operate through a range of fundamental distinctions, like the ones between body and mind, object and subject, is and ought, fact and value, and nature and culture. Science, often written in the singular, is about discovering matters of fact about a preexistent, natural, and material world, about which entities exist in the world, how they relate to each other, and how we can intervene to bring about change. On the other side of the divide, we locate the seat of self-governing (autonomous) subjects in the deep internal space of the human mind. Although we know from elementary human anatomy that there is no empty space in the skull, we have come to understand ourselves as inhabiting this private internal space. This nonmaterial space of the mind is coextensive with autobiographical consciousness and shaped by biography and experience [9]. This idea underlies the important humanist notions of personhood and human agency. I have called both psychology's internal space of the human mind and the modern notion of the autonomous, human subject for *irreal* to express the ambiguousness in two senses in which we think about ourselves: (1) the sense that we are coextensive with our body, with the entailment that the "I" or "Self" ends with the disintegration of the body/brain, and (2) the sense that there is something more, something that is separate and distinct from our body/brain, an immaterial entity (soul?) that we perhaps hope will live on after death [10]. Obviously, this notion of the human subject is also a key concept in ethical reasoning. Autobiographical consciousness is the defining feature of what makes us living human beings. It is called *autobiographical* because it locates the current self in a temporal continuum of a lived past (memory functions) and an anticipated but open future (functions of planning and evaluation of alternative courses of action) [11]. The evolutionary emergence of autobiographical consciousness produced, most notably in humans, the awareness that we all, at some future time, will die. *Memento mori!* It also produced the anticipation of suffering that has not yet come to pass. Entities that have developed or have the *potential* to develop an autobiographical consciousness in their deep internal space are the subjects of ethical care, worthy of ethical and legal protection without discrimination by other human beings and society. The possession of that potential capacity is, in an essentialist understanding of medical ethics, necessary and sufficient to qualify for ethical and legal protection. A fully developed autobiographical consciousness provides its owner with the possibility of choice, subject to its own and society's laws instead of the deterministic laws of nature. The laws of nature and the laws of man are separate matters.

Hence, we conceive of the deep, internal, private space of the individual mind as being coextensive with consciousness and with the operative agent doing the intending, willing, emoting, conceptualizing, and associating of concepts to language that we associate with thinking. It is the thinking that we do in this internal space, and of which we are consciously aware, that we have come to define reductively as human cognition. To define something is a process or activity of *delineating*, of tracing a boundary that simultaneously produces an inside and an outside, that what belongs and that which is excluded. Although produced in real time in the same brain, emotions and feelings have no place in what has become the epitome of human cognition: rational thinking and reasoning. This conception of the rational human subject not only disembodied cognition, displacing the body but also displaced emotions as a form of cognition, that is, as the human body's principal biological valuation system. It is in such a "space of representation," featuring a fundamental distinction between objective facts and subjective values, between reasoning and feeling, that traditional forms of medical-ethical reasoning gain traction; get the facts straight before moving on to sorting out the moral quandaries and dilemmas. It is such a space that makes the idea that end-of-life decision-making should be informed by medical knowledge about a patient's disease, treatment possibilities, results, and prognoses seem persuasive and right.

Recent work in the neurosciences challenges the distinction between detached, rational reasoning occurring in the bark of the cerebral hemispheres (higher brain functions) and emotions generated in specialized, lower areas of the midbrain. Effectively, this work reclaims emotions for the appropriate understanding of all forms of biological, embodied cognition

[11–13]. Embodied cognition biologists argue that cognition is a fundamental feature of biological life [14–16]. Cognition is a function that emerges with the formation of a living organism. Cognition is coextensive with the recursive sensorimotor loops of the embodied activity of living organisms. Life = embodied action = cognition. The repeated, recursive cycles of action and perception constitute an intentional arc. Intentionality is here conceived as an organism's orientedness toward its socionatural environment. The Self is, in this view, the result of ongoing, here-and-now dynamic biological processes in a brain that is in continuous interaction with the body in which it is embedded and with the body's physical and social environment. This is also the pre-position on which my own arguments in this paper are built: all judgments about the world, about human nature, and core human values are the products of *cognitive* recursive processes embedded in the bodies, brains, and activities of individuals and the recursive interactions among and practices of members of *collectives*. Damasio argues that the cognizing Self is "a perpetually recreated neurobiological state" [17]. Arguing along the same lines, we could say that the worlds of cognizing, meaning-making collectives are the emergent outcomes of perpetually recreated discursive-material practices [18]. Another way of saying this is that sciences do not *represent* a separate, pre-existent world, but that sciences conceived as collective sociomaterial practices *perform* the phenomena that make up the world we live and die in. They form, to use Latour's term, our "modes of existence" [19]. Within such formations, there is no a priori separation between what is, what we know about what is, and what we value and care about. If there seem to be such fundamental distinctions, then they are the result of the work of philosophers (of science, of mind, etc.) being appropriated by scientists into the onto-epistemological foundation of their science. These processes can and should be studied empirically. The social study of "knowledge practices" is concerned with the ways sociomaterial "modes of ordering" come into being and with the power involved in that process. Multiple modes of ordering (plural) exist simultaneously; sometimes going comfortably together, giving rise to frictions and oppositions at other times and places [3].

## 3. Conceptual blending and modes of ordering

Cognitive linguists George Lakoff and Mark Johnson have long recognized the embodied nature of cognition [20–22]. Studying everyday and scientific language, they demonstrated that our understanding of the world, as it is expressed through language, is imbued with metaphorical imagery inferred from our embodied experience. The basic idea is that our embodied being and acting in the world provides the metaphorical schemas that constitute language and human understanding. An example is our basic understanding of causal relationships and human agency rooted in our embodied experience of pushing or moving objects around and observing the effects of that action. In a similar sense, our understanding of being emotionally moved is rooted in the experience of an outside force being applied to our bodies. We understand the passage of time metaphorically as a movement through space, a notion that is materially anchored in analogue clocks [23]. We may understand dying, a passage from one state into another, as involving a passage through space, a journey across the water and into the west, to undying lands, or from this earthly place full of suffering to a sacred, heavenly place of peace and tranquility where we will meet again those loved ones that passed before us. Death itself is often understood through militant metaphors as an enemy that must be fought off. But death may also be understood metaphorically as a welcome friend that saves us from further suffering in this world, or as a pre-emptive escape from the intolerable, meaningless, empty days ahead. The basic operation that a metaphor performs is one of mapping, of the transfer or projection of entities, processes and structure from a *source* domain to a *target* domain. Metaphorical schemas combine to build complex and abstract conceptual understandings.

Gilles Fauconnier and Mark Turner take Lakoff and Johnson's work further and develop it into a theory of conceptual blending [2, 4–7]. Metaphorical mapping is only one form of conceptual blending. There are several more. Conceptual blending can be schematically presented by way of a minimal network that comprises at least three mental spaces: at least two input mental spaces and the blending space [2]. The input spaces selectively contribute or project structure and elements to the blended space in which these are integrated. Structure and elements that occupy analogous positions in the two input spaces, which in other words map between domains, may be compressed into identity and human scale. Conceptual blends can be elaborated by further blending with input spaces that already are blends. Biologists, for example, have blended the evolutionary history of life on earth with the developmental history of an individual from conception to birth and into adulthood, giving rise to the (problematic) idea that ontogeny recapitulates phylogeny [24]. Neuroscientists have blended the sequential emergence in biological organisms of what Damasio calls a proto-, core- and autobiographical-consciousness with the macroanatomy of the brain, associating proto-consciousness with the brainstem—that we share with animals, core consciousness with the midbrain—that we share with closer animal relatives that we assume not to be self-conscious yet, and specifically human autobiographical consciousness with the phylogenetically newest neocortex of the large hemispheres [10, 11].

In many instances of conceptual blending, one or more of the input spaces is already a blended space. Mark Turner calls the blends that result from blending spaces that already are blends for *hyper-blends*. Many of our most treasured ideas concerning human beings are hyper-blends, like the notion of an autonomous human agent inhabiting a nonmaterial deep internal space inside our skull. In conceptual blending theory, it is not only analogies and similarities that matter, but dis-analogies are also important, including their either problematic or productive entailments. The notion of brain death, for example, is a hyper-blend, blending the idea of the legally certified death of a person with diagnostic procedures proving in a warm, breathing, and heart-beating body that the brain is irreversibly damaged. The dis-analogies between common notions and experiences of a dead person (as cold, nonbreathing, and with no puls) and the warm, heart-beating brain dead patient can be hard to accommodate for next of kin. The productive entailment of the brain death hyper-blend is that good quality donor-organs can legally be extirpated for transplantation purposes without running the risk of being prosecuted for murder.

Furthermore, conceptual blending is conducive to counterfactual reasoning. The input spaces to a blend do not have to factually exist. They may be counterfactual. In some cases, the counterfactual space does not even carry with it the suggestion that it might be possible. In many other cases, the counterfactual space implies a state or a scenario that may be possible but that has not yet come to pass. In the chronological/biological age hyper-blend, the discrepancy between a person's biological age—calculated by measuring biological indicators of aging—and chronological age entails a counterfactual scenario of premature death. The responsible self-management of modifiable risk factors can prevent this scenario. The premature death scenario will remain counterfactual unless you take care, take responsibility for your own health. The point is not that the blend is a "possible world" or a true representation of the world, but that the blend suggests alternative ways of engaging with the world, and whose primary responsibility that is.

The power a particular hyper-blend can hold over people, fueling its own protection and the rejection of alternatives, should not be underestimated. Apparently, this is the case when deeply engrained beliefs about our own human nature, living and dying are challenged. Conceptual blending is not just some language game that we can enter into and get out of at will. Conceptual blending is part and parcel of the discursive-material practices that are constitutive for and order the world in which we live. We live in the blend! But neither should we neglect the contingency, multiplicity, diversity, and simultaneous coexistence of different modes of ordering life and the world, and how they relate to and interfere with each other. "For," Mol and Law argue, "the various modes of ordering, logics, styles, practices, and the realities they perform do not exist in isolation from one another ... They are not islands unto themselves, closed cultures, self-contained paradigms, or bubbles. [T]hey interfere with one another and reveal ... partial connections." "Often," Mol and Law continue, "it is not so much a matter of living in a single mode of ordering or of 'choosing' between them. Rather it is that we find ourselves at places where these modes join. Somewhere in the interferences something crucial happens ... complexity is created, emerging where various modes of ordering (styles, logics) come together and add up comfortably or in tension, or both" [3].

## 4. A blended space for moral arguments: the balance sheet

As an embodied cognitive operation, *judging* is a matter of *balancing* and of weighing one against the other. Take one object in your left hand and a second object in your right hand: Which one weighs the most? This idea of judgment as a balancing act is materially anchored in the weighing instrument called a *balance*. We also use *balancing* in the sense of *re-balancing*, of re-establishing equality of "weight" between two entities when that balance has been disturbed. An eye for an eye, a tooth for a tooth! The proportional retribution balances the harm received. Justice is done. Justice is re-established. The image of the *balance* has been blended into the iconography of our legal system, together with the blindfold (impartiality) and the sword (punishment, retribution).

In economic practices, the blend of the *balance* has been elaborated with calculative features. The *balance sheet* is an archetypical space designed for the display and calculation of *proportional* relationships between costs and benefits, gains and losses, debts and possessions, and debit and credit. Balance sheets allow for forms of what Winther-Jørgensen calls for *strong calculation*, that is, forms of calculation where the end result can be expressed as a numerical number [25]. The numerical values in which judgments based on strong calculations are expressed have strong appeal for policy makers and politicians. However, not all forms of balance sheet calculation are strong. Many are weak. Moral judgments are often of this kind. The familiar expression "on the balance of it"—followed by a decision or conclusion, that is a judgment—is a marker of some form of preceding calculation, strong or weak, that involves the weighing of factual states and counterfactual possibilities, probabilities, and proportionalities, against each other.

Foster provides a telling example of how the balance sheet is used in moral reasoning and judgment [26]. The case is one in which there is a dispute about what is in the patient's best interest. Some cases go to court. In a legal setting, Foster explains: "If it is to mean anything – if it is to be real – it has to be procedurally entrenched" [26]. The reasoning goes like this:

**a.** Human life is sacred. A corollary of that is that it must be a presumption that it is in the patient's best interest to continue to live.

**b.** The presumption can be rebutted.

**c.** What is required to rebut is evidence that continued existence would be intolerable (the so-called intolerability test).

An appellate court judge explains how such an *intolerability test* should be executed.

> The first instance judge with the responsibility to make an evaluation of the best interest of the claimant lacking capacity should draw up a *balance sheet*. The first entrance should be any factor or factors of actual benefit. Then on the other sheet, the judge should write any counter-balancing dis-benefits to the applicant. Then the judge should enter on each sheet the potential gains and losses in each instance making some estimate of the extent of the possibility that the gain or loss might accrue. At the end of the exercise the judge should be better placed to *strike a balance* between the sum of the certain and possible gains against the sum of the certain and possible losses. Obviously, only if the *account* is in relatively significant credit will the judge conclude that the application is likely to advance the best interest of the claimant [26] (my italics).

In the case of the intolerability test, the judge who performs the calculations in the balance sheet cannot do this on the basis of events that have already been experienced, but he must to a large extent rely on estimates of counterfactual events and experiences that have not yet come to pass. Furthermore, there may be limitations on what kinds of suffering or relief can enter the calculation.

## 5. Suffering as the common currency on personal end-of-life balance sheets

Suffering is a common currency on the costs side of end-of-life balance sheets. On the other benefits side of the balance sheet, suffering is balanced by more time of life, but not at any cost. The balance sheet can be a seriously ill or dying person's personal dilemma to figure out what to do and how to proceed. Think of a patient with an advanced form of cancer. This is the familiar quandary that follows from the uncertainty that you cannot know in advance whether the extra time of life that life-prolonging treatment will give has a quality of life that is worth living. Do the good days on which you have time to live outweigh the bad days that are filled with suffering? Shall I accept the offer of life-prolonging treatment at the cost of prolonged suffering? Or shall I accept that death is imminent and use the time left to settle my affairs and say farewell to next of kin and loved ones?

One gets the impression that the expected answer is obvious: Of course, you must choose for more time of life, to be with your partner, to see your children grow up and hold a newborn grandchild in your arms. But is this choice so obvious?

In affluent countries with advanced health care systems, cancer treatment has been centralized in cancer clinics associated with university hospitals, combining research and teaching with treatment and patient care. In these hospitals, clinicians also hold research and teaching positions in the associated university. Through their professional organizations, these professors in oncology may be involved in the elaboration of professional guidelines for the diagnosis and treatment of particular forms of cancer. Many patients attending the clinic for diagnostics and treatment are enrolled in research protocols that are part of international, collaborative multicenter studies [27]. Today, these studies do not compare cancer treatment with the natural course of the disease under nontreatment. They compare slightly different multimodal treatment options with already existing ones. The by far most important effect variable is *survival* in one or other form, as duration of remission, mean time to relapse, or mean time to death. In these centers, quite aggressive treatments of even advanced stages of cancer have become the default treatment option offered to patients. "We will fight together!" one patient information brochure exclaims, suggesting simultaneously an expectation that the patient also fights her cancer [28]. There is a particular notion of *courage* here. The kind of courage the patient must muster to suffer through the ordeals of surgical, radiation, and chemotherapy to win more time of life to spend with her children and spouse, and to help medicine become better at treating cancer and, hence, safe future lives. Cancer centers are in the business of adding and maximizing survival. Perhaps it should come as no surprise that the alternative, accepting that death is imminent and entering into a palliative trajectory, requiring a different kind of courage, is not always offered to patients in these centers [28].

Aggressive treatment and refusing life-prolonging treatment are two different trajectories that exhibit path dependency. Once you have entered into one or the other, it is difficult to go back. The suffering endured under treatment is the investment a patient must make to gain more time of life. To make it worthwhile, the good days must balance the bad days. When bad days outnumber good days, counting and summarizing days of each kind will not be sufficient. It may be necessary to increase the value of each good day, of each moment with your children or grandchildren to make the sum of them balance out and surpass the costs.

We should, furthermore, consider to what extent the treatment regime contributes to an increase of suffering. As diagnostic technologies make it possible to achieve the goal of early and even presymptomatic diagnosis of cancers, the suffering a patient endures is induced to an increasing degree by the treatment. Much of the suffering is iatrogenic and not caused by the disease.

Keating and Cambrioso argue that the evolution and history of cancer after the Second World War is the evolution of the disease under specific treatment regimens. It is a treatment history rather than a "natural history" [27]. Systemic cancer treatment intervenes in the biology of the disease. Today, it is more apparent than ever that cancer is not only a *clonal* disease, meaning that the origin of cancer cells can be traced back to a first, single cancerous ancestral cell that, having acquired the capacity of limitless cell division, gives rise to limitless numbers of descendants. Cancer is also *adaptive*. Or as Mukherjee puts it, cancer is a clonally *evolving* disease [29]. Due to some degree of genetic instability, every generation of cancer cells creates a small number of cells that are genetically different from their parents. With each volley of chemotherapeutic drugs that does not kill all cancer cells, a few mutant clones that can resist the assault grow out. In Mukherjee's *clonal selection cancer blend*, blending the course of a disease in a patient with the evolutionary history of life forms on earth, "[t]his mirthless, relentless cycle of mutation, selection and overgrowth generates cells that are more and more adapted to survival and growth … Cancer thus exploits the fundamental logic of evolution unlike any other illness. If we, as a species, are the ultimate product of Darwinian selection, then so, too, is this incredible disease that lurks inside us" [29]. In a sense, the "war on cancer" is a war on life itself.

Cancer treatment regimens *coproduce* the disease phases of *remission* and *relapse*. As the apparatus of collaborative groups matured, clinical trials targeted specific disease phases: trials for initial treatment, trials for first remission, trials for relapse, and so on. The disease at relapse was no longer the same as the disease initially diagnosed, requiring new drugs or new drug combinations. Without chemotherapeutic treatment regimens, these phases would not exist.

For the individual patient, cancer treatment regimens produce the protracted courses of disease, including the harm done to patients as a result of the "all-out assault" nature of the treatment that so many present-day cancer patients go through. The suffering caused by the treatment can be far greater and protracted than the suffering caused by the disease itself. It is a high price patients pay.

## 6. The balance sheets of euthanasia and palliative sedation

The figure of the balance sheet of suffering is also apparent in arguments policing the distinction between euthanasia and assisted suicide on one hand and palliative sedation on the other [30]. These are arguments not only about the implications of the intolerability of suffering but also about what kind of items are allowed onto the balance sheet and which are not.

Palliative sedation is described as the intentional pharmacological reduction of the patient's consciousness with the aim to reduce intolerable suffering from intractable physical symptoms that cannot be managed otherwise. Palliative sedation until death is considered to be a last-resort option. Proponents of palliative sedation in end-of-life care take great care to present palliative sedation as an ordinary, medical treatment that is different in kind from euthanasia.

Palliative sedation is provided with the intention to relief suffering, with an explicit focus on the *intention* with which the treatment is given. Often within the same sentence, under the same breath, it is added that the *intention* is not to hasten death. We encounter this figure in many variations. Of course, in this blend, the intent to hasten death would be equivalent to euthanasia or physician assisted suicide. The blend is further elaborated by blending with moral or legal positions. Depending on one's moral conviction or on the jurisdiction in which one works, hastening a patient's death would be equivalent with murder. An international panel of expert clinicians reviewing the literature on palliative sedation in the last weeks of life concluded that

> The decision to offer sedation to relieve intolerable suffering during the last weeks of life presents no distinct ethical problem, provided that there is *no intention* to hasten death. It is distinct from euthanasia because (a) it has the *intention* to provide symptom relief, (b) it is a proportionate intervention and (c) the death of the patient is not a criterion for the success of the treatment [31] (my *emphasis*).

In medical treatment, there is always a risk of detrimental effects, but these are unintended side effects. In one general medical or pharmacological sense, *proportionality* refers to the due care requirement that the level of sedation should not be deeper than is necessary to alleviate distress and suffering. When mild sedation (somnolence; a form of reduction of consciousness from which one can be aroused through appropriate forms of stimulation) achieves the intended result, then one should not aim for deep sedation (from which one cannot be aroused) [31]. In end-of-life care, severe anxiety is treated with sedatives from the same family of substances as those used in palliative sedation. *Proportionality* of anxiety treatment may require a dosage to be increased to levels where reduction of consciousness occurs as an *unintended side effect*. However, when the intention was not to expressly produce unconsciousness, or so the argument goes, this would not constitute palliative sedation.

When intentions *cause* actions, the reverse should also apply, that is, that intentions can be backtracked from the records in which action patterns and the traces that these leave behind are documented.

> The *intention* of PST [= Palliative Sedation Treatment] can be *assessed by the proportionality …* of the action. *Intent may be judged* by looking at the drug record. Repeated doses, titrated to ease an individual's distress, are the *mark* of proportionated sedation. Single large doses are the *mark* of ignorance and intentional harm [31] (my *emphasis*).

Cases in which there is a covert intention to hasten death through high dosages of sedatives constitute "covert euthanasia" or "euthanasia by stealth" (relief of suffering *by* death). The words "covert" and "stealth" place these ways of doing end-of-life care on the wrong side of the border, morally and legally. Future suffering relieved or prevented *by* death is not allowed on the benefit side of this balance sheet of suffering.

The Norwegian guidelines for palliative sedation to the dying, published in 2001 by the Norwegian Medical Association, provide a telling example of how suffering relieved by death is excluded from the balance sheet [32]. Against the claim that euthanasia contributes to the relief of suffering, the Norwegian guidelines for palliative sedation to the dying argue that suffering belongs to life and life experience.

> Talk about the absence or relief of something that belongs to life is meaningless when the patient is dead. ... A sedated patient is without suffering, but simultaneously with life experience. Yet, it makes sense to say that suffering has been relieved, because the patient still lives and can be woken again. [32]

At least the potential for life experience is still present. The Norwegian guidelines dismiss the counterfactual argument that says that "not-living-anymore" will stop further suffering from occurring, although this is, in another blend, obviously true.

In Norway, suffering that has been prevented by the patient's death is inadmissible as an entry into the balance sheet of human suffering. Positions on ethical, legal, and medical issues, on probabilities and causal relationships have been crafted together in a coherent framework that both shapes and restricts choices available to dying patients and next-of-kin?

Contrary to Norway, the Netherlands have carved out another path that goes deeper into the borderland of life and death. Historically, the Dutch physicians who, together with their patients, pioneered the practice of euthanasia in the Netherlands defended their actions with an appeal to the appeal the patients' suffering made on their moral duty to not abandon but to help them [33]. The Netherlands allow patients to ask for more active termination of life to prevent suffering, simultaneously allowing physicians to grant such a request when they perceive it their never easy duty to provide assistance in dying when live can no longer be saved or prolonged. *Suffering prevented by death* is allowed as an entry on the benefit side of the end-of-life balance sheet. Safeguards marking that path, that is subject to the Dutch Penal Code, in the form of due care requirements, are consequently tougher than those for palliative sedation. These due care requirements include a second opinion by another physician, compulsory notification of each case to a review committee, and in each case a decision of exemption from prosecution and punishment. "The offence ... shall not be punishable if it has been committed by a physician who has met the requirements of due care ..." (Article 293 of the Dutch Penal Code, as amended by the law of 2001) [33].

## 7. Suffering from life

It is possible to specify the differences between items allowed to be entered on the balance sheet even further. In Norway, euthanasia and assisted suicide are illegal. But even in its guidelines for palliative sedation in end-of-life care the Norwegian Medical Association is very restrictive. In its 2001 guidelines, it is only intolerable and refractory *physical* symptoms that can provide a proper medical indication for the intended, proportional pharmaceutical reduction of the patient's consciousness, and therewith life experience. Mental symptoms are not allowed on that balance sheet [32]. The Norwegian Medical Association revised its guidelines for palliative sedation in 2014 [34]. It maintains its position that palliative sedation is a last-resort option; a treatment that, although ordinary and legal, should only be given in exceptional cases of intolerable suffering resulting from or dominated by physical symptoms. However, the 2014 guidelines provide a small opening toward mental suffering by stating that "psychological symptoms alone are only in rare cases indication for palliative sedation" [34]. In a paper in the Medical Association's journal, these psychological symptoms are specified as "serious and treatment refractory psychological symptoms and delirium with extreme unrest and confusion, provided that first an attempt has been made to correct pathophysiolocal causes" [35]. These are mental symptoms associated with the process of dying.

The Dutch law regulating euthanasia and assisted suicide makes no distinction between physical and mental suffering, including suffering from psychiatric conditions like schizophrenia or bipolar disease. There is recognition that the mental suffering from psychiatric conditions over long time, and without the prospect of improvement, can induce in patients the wish to die. Dutch law has made it possible for these patients to ask for and receive professional help in ending their lives on request, provided proper procedures and due care requirements are followed.

Starting in the early 1990s, in the Netherlands, there is currently an ongoing discussion about the question whether the kind of suffering that should be allowed as entries on the balance sheet should be expanded beyond psychiatric conditions to include *suffering from life*. In 2010, a group of publicly well-known former politicians, physicians, university professors, journalists, and artists established the Out of Free Will civil initiative, *Uit Vrije Wil*, working toward the legalization of professional help to die for people of old age who consider their live *completed* [36]. The people this concerns are people who have reached respectable ages of 75 or older and who have developed a sustained wish to die. They do not want to have to keep on living a life that has become meaningless and without prospect. They may or may not suffer from the accumulated physical symptoms of common ailments that come with old age, but that is not the source of their wish to die. The reasons they give for their wish to die vary but have often to do with the loss of next of kin and spouses; the feeling of not being needed anymore after having lived an active and fruitful life, of being sidelined by society; a fear of loosing their independence; of becoming dependent on others; the lack of meaningful everyday life activities. Life itself, or better, the prospect of living through the many empty and meaningless days ahead has become the source of a kind of existential suffering [37]. Some of them still have a partner they live with or adult children with families, and they enjoy spending time with them. But on the balance of it, these moments do not outweigh the burden they suffer from having lost the prospect of a meaningful future. They are, to use Wijngaarden´s phrase, "incurably old."

The issue of legalization of professional help to die to old age people who consider their life completed was brought up in parliament during the 2014 evaluation of the Dutch law on euthanasia and assisted suicide. The government commissioned an advisory report on the issue from a group of experts. The committee concluded that the extant legal framework already provides sufficient possibilities for this presumably small group of people. Hence, it is not advisable to allow, with regard to assisted suicide, more freedom to emerge than is already provided by the current legal framework [38]. Despite this conclusion, in the year preceding the parliamentary elections of March 2017, several liberal parties expressed their support for an expansion of the law and include the suffering from having to live on as a legitimate ground for asking but also receiving professional help in ending one's life. In 2016, member of parliament for the liberal democratic party D´66, Pia Dijkstra, prepared and submitted a bill to this effect, arguing that the freedom of every citizen to shape and live their lives in accordance with their own preferences also includes decisions concerning the final phase and the end of life. Everyone has the right to leave this life, or conversely, no one is obliged to keep on living [39]. Forcing someone to continue living a life that has become meaningless not only violates this person's right to self-determination, but it also constitutes a form of harm. It should not be a crime to help!

It is uncertain whether the bill will pass the next parliament, and of course, there is an opposition, not only from religious parties in parliament but also from mental health professionals, arguing that these people are mentally ill, suffering from a detachment syndrome. They should receive treatment not be given assistance to die.

## 8. Human rights as currency on end-of-life balance sheets: patient autonomy vs. professional conscience

In the previous sections, a different type of balance sheet has been lurking: the balance sheet that sets up and weighs the patient's right to self-determination against health professional's right to conscience.

The Norwegian 2001 guidelines on palliative sedation to the dying explicitly require *proportionality* between the severity of the patient's suffering and the moral gravity of the demand put to a physician. To ask a physician to collaborate in the permanent reduction of a patient's consciousness, and therewith life experience, is of such significance that this can only be requested in cases where the patient's suffering is of equal magnitude [30, 32].

The concern for health professionals' right to conscience is also evident in these and other guidelines' preoccupation with the *cause of death*. Or rather, their preoccupation with avoiding that a palliative intervention can be perceived as a contributing causal factor to the death of the patient. After the patient's death, it is the underlying disease that should stand alone as the cause of death. Graef and Dean wrote that "[t]he desired outcome of PST is symptom relief and a peaceful, quiet death *by the natural course of the disease*" [31] (my italics). Note that the causal relationship is signified by the word "by." The agent causing death is the disease. Note also that the quote ignores that modern medicine has transformed the courses of many diseases through myriad of interventions and attempts to cure or delay the disease so that it is no longer possible to talk about the *natural* course of a disease. To a large extent, modern medicine has *chronified* the diseases it cannot cure [40]. The word "natural" must here be understood in opposition to artificial or "caused by a medical intervention." On the question whether palliative sedation has an impact on the exact time of death, Dutch guidelines conclude that, when administered proportionally, palliative sedation does not hasten death. The Norwegian guidelines are not satisfied with the level of evidence for this conclusion and argue that "even though it is claimed that palliative sedation does not foreshorten life, it can never be completely ruled out that a patient dies as a result of the sedation." The risk of this happening increases *proportionally* with the time the patient spends in an unconscious or sedated condition [32].

Both the patient and the doctor or the nurse have a right to autonomy and self-determination that derives from the same Universal Declaration of Human Rights concerning the right to freedom of thought, conscience, and religion. So, on the balance of it, whose autonomy shall carry the most weight in end-of-life decision making?

## 9. Consequences of restrictive end-of-life care policies for the balance sheet of suffering

The same figure of the balance sheet of suffering and human rights is used in both countries, but it is operated quite differently. Norway is the more restrictive of the two countries, at least in its policy documents, laws, and professional guidelines. It puts more constraints on both dying patients and physicians and other health professionals. The Netherlands have developed more generous end-of-life care practices, allowing patients to ask for more active termination of life at the patient's explicit and sustained request.

The notion of constraints can be understood in two different ways. A common understanding of a constraint is that of a prohibition, an arrangement that aims to prevent something from happening. The other understanding of a constraint puts emphasis on the channeling effects of constraints, the way in which a dam in a river, for example, channels the water current into a tube to produce hydropower energy. Or the ways in which environmental constraints can channel the direction of emergent biological forms (volleys of chemotherapy impacting the biology of the cancer; the wide spread use of antibiotics producing multiresistant bacteria). Could the strong emphasis on the sanctity of life in palliative end-of-life care in fact increase the amount and duration of suffering in dying patients? Of course, this is a question that is difficult to answer. But, I will argue, there are indications that this might be the case.

One reason is apparent in the definitions that palliative sedation has received in Norwegian guidelines. As a last resort option, palliative sedation is defined as the intentional, pharmacological reduction of the patient's consciousness with the aim to reduce intolerable suffering from intractable *physical* symptoms that cannot be managed otherwise. Suffering from intractable physical symptoms is a proper medical indication. Suffering from psychiatric condition is not allowed onto the Norwegian balance sheet of suffering. Depending on the degree of physicians' compliance with these professional guidelines one can argue that there may be suffering that is addressed too late, and perhaps insufficiently out of fear for being accused of euthanasia.

When definitions of palliative care are provided, the definition is more often than not followed, under the same breath, by the reassurance that palliative care/palliation does not hasten death nor prolong it. As a factual statement, this must be false. Palliative treatment affects the temporal dimensions of dying. However, the evaluation of a palliative treatment's effect on the timing of death is different depending on its direction, whether the process of dying is accelerated or delayed. Even a small change toward an earlier death is viewed with suspicion, because the *intention* of palliative care is not to hasten death or relief suffering by death. At the end of the day, it is the underlying disease, and it alone, that must stand out as the agent responsible for the death of the patient. Unfortunately, this preoccupation with avoiding that *acts of care* can be construed as causal co-factors to the death of a dying patient induces uncertainty, anxiety, and feelings of guilt in both health professionals and next of kin. A shift in the timing of death in the other direction, delaying the process of dying, is valued differently, because it gives the patient more time and more life experience. However, more time as a result of palliative treatment also allows the erosion of body and mind to become deeper before death finally arrives.

## 10. Conclusion

In many western countries with highly developed health care systems, the law of the land has delegated the *competence* to make end-of-life care decisions to physicians, based on the assumption that these are medical decisions that require knowledge and expertise about treatment possibilities, documented results, and prognosis. The medical-professional literature describes the point at which life-prolonging treatment is no longer possible and its transition into a palliative trajectory as a *medical assessment and decision*. Despite the fact that respect for the patient's autonomy is first among the four principles of medical ethics, in practice, our autonomy is constrained at a time when it perhaps matters most, at the time of our dying [10]. I am not advocating that patients facing death "put in the oars"—as the Norwegian saying goes—too early. When they do, they may spend a long time waiting for death. However, I would support people reclaiming important aspects of end-of-life decision making from medicine, give priority to their own versions of the balance sheet of their lives and values, and achieve or maintain a greater degree of direction over the manner, place, and timing of death.

## Acknowledgements

The article processing charges for this chapter have been funded by a grant from the open access publication fund of UiT The Arctic University of Norway.

## Author details

Ger Wackers

Address all correspondence to: ger.wackers@uit.no

UiT The Arctic University of Norway, Institute for Health and Care Sciences, Campus Narvik, Norway

## References

[1] Rheinberger H-J. An Epistemology of the Concrete. Twentieth-Century Histories of Life. Durham: Duke University Press; 2010

[2] Turner M. The Origin of Ideas. Blending, Creativity, and the Human Spark. Oxford: Oxford University Press; 2014

[3] Law J, Mol A, editors. Complexities. Social Studies of Knowledge Practices. Durham & London: Duke University Press; 2002

[4] Fauconnier G. Mental Spaces. Aspects of Meaning Construction in Natural Language. Cambridge: Cambridge University Press; 1994

[5] Fauconnier G. Mappings in Thought and Language. Cambridge, UK: Cambridge University Press; 1997

[6] Fauconnier G, Turner M. The Way We Think. Conceptual Blending and the Mind's Hidden Complexities. New York: Basic Books; 2002

[7] Turner M. Cognitive Dimensions of Social Science. The Way We Think About Politics, Economics, Law and Society. Oxford: Oxford University Press; 2001

[8] Coulson S. Semantic Leaps. Frame-Shifting and Conceptual Blending in Meaning Construction. Cambridge: Cambridge University Press; 2001

[9] Rose N, Abi-Rached J. Neuro: The New Brain Sciences and the Management of the Mind. Princeton: Princeton University Press; 2013

[10] Wackers G. Truncated autonomy. Neocortical selves, reverse reductionism and end-of-life care. In: Clark P, editor. Bioethics—Medical, Ethical and Legal Perspectives. Rijeka: InTech; 2016. pp. 181-198; http://dx.doi.org/10.5772/66044

[11] Damasio A. Self Comes to Mind. Constructing the Conscious Brain. New York: Pantheon Books; 2010

[12] Panksepp J, Biven L. The Archaeology of Mind: Neuroevolutionary Origins of Human Emotions. New York: W.W. Norton & Company; 2012

[13] Pessoa L. The Cognitive-Emotional Brain. From Interactions to Integration. Cambridge, MA: The MIT Press; 2013

[14] Varela FJ, Thompson E, Rosch E. The Embodied Mind. Cognitive Science and Human Experience. Cambridge, MA.: The MIT Press; 1993

[15] Freeman WJ. How Brains Make Up Their Minds. New York: Columbia University Press; 2000

[16] Núñez R, Freeman WJ, editors. Reclaiming Cognition: The Primacy of Action, Intention and Emotion. Thorverton, UK: Imprint Academic; 2000

[17] Damasio A. Descartes' Error. Emotion, Reason, and the Human Brain. New York: Penguin Books; 1994

[18] Barad K. Meeting the Universe Halfway. Quantum Physics and the Entanglement of Matter and Meaning. Durham: Duke University Press; 2007

[19] Latour B. An Inquiry into Modes of Existence. An Anthropology of the Moderns. Cambridge, MA.: Harvard University Press; 2013

[20] Lakoff G, Johnson M. Metaphors We Live By. Chicago: The University of Chicago Press; 1980

[21] Johnson M. The Body in the Mind. The Bodily Basis of Meaning, Imagination, and Reason. Chicago: University of Chicago Press; 1987

[22] Lakoff G, Johnson M. Philosophy in the Flesh. The Embodied Mind and its Challenge to Western Thought. New York: Basic Books; 1999

[23] Hutchins E. Cognition in the Wild. Cambridge, MA: The MIT Press; 1995

[24] Gould SJ. Ontogeny and Phylogeny. Cambridge, MA: The Belknap Press of Harvard University Press; 1977

[25] Winther Jørgensen M. Patient-centered decision making? Biomedicine between evidence-based medicine and self-determination. Evidence & Policy. 2015;11(3):311-329

[26] Foster C. Choosing Life, Choosing Death. The Tyranny of Autonomy in Medical Ethics and Law. Oxford and Portland, Oregon: Hart Publishing; 2009

[27] Keating P, Cambrosio A. Cancer on Trial: Oncology as a New Style of Practice. Chicago and London: The University of Chicago Press; 2012

[28] Wackers G. Recursive health care structures and choice in the manner of our dying: An autoethnographic account. Qualitative Health Research. 2015;26(4):452 - 465. DOI: 10.1177/1049732315576498

[29] Mukherjee S. The Emperor of All Maladies. A Biography of Cancer. New York: Scribner; 2010

[30] Wackers G. Into the wild country: Epistemic issues in professional guidelines for palliative sedation in end-of-life care. Evidence & Policy. 2015;11(3):331-349

[31] de Graeff A, Dean M. Palliative sedation therapy in the last weeks of life: A literature review and recommendations for standards. Journal of Palliative Medicine. 2007; 10(1):67-85

[32] Dnl [Den norske legeforening]. Retningslinjer for lindrende sedering til døende. Oslo: Den norske legeforening, Rådet for legeetikk; 2001. [Guidelines for palliative sedation to the dying. The Norwegian Medical Association/Council for Medical Ethics]. Available from: http:77www.legeforeningen.no/id/3942

[33] ten Have H, Welie J. Death and Medical Power: An Ethical Analysis of Dutch Euthanasia Practice. Maidenhead: Open University Press; 2005

[34] Dnl [Den norske legeforening]. Rettningslinjer for lindrende sedering i livets sluttfase. Oslo: Den norske legeforening; 2014. [Palliative sedation in life's final phase. The Norwegian Medical Association]

[35] Førde R, Materstvedt LJ, Markestad T, Kongsgaard UE, von Hofacker S, Brelin S, Ore S, Laudal M. Lindrende sedering i livets sluttfase—reviderte retningslinjer. Tidsskr Nor Legeforen. 2015;135(3):220-221. [Palliative sedation in life's final phase—revised guidelines]

[36] Uit Vrije Wil. Burgerinitiatief voltooid leven. URL: uitvrije wil.nu (Accessed April 30, 2017). [Out of Free Wil. Civil initiative completed life]

[37] van Wijngaarden E. Voltooid leven. Over leven en willen sterven. Amsterdam: Atlas Contact; 2016. [Completed life. On living and wanting to die]

[38] Schnabel P, et al. Voltooid leven. Over hulp bij zelfdoding aan mensen die hun leven voltooid achten. Den Haag: Adviescommissie voltooid leven; 2016. [Completed life. On assisted suicide for people who deem their life completed. Advisory Committee Completed Life]

[39] Dijkstra P. Voorstel van wet van het lid Pia Dijkstra houdende toetsing van levensbeeindiging van ouderen op verzoek. Den Haag: Memorie van toelichting; 2016. [Bill of law from member (of parliament) Pia Dijkstra concerning the assessment of termination of life of elderly on demand. Explanatory memorandum]

[40] Pols J. The Chronofication of Illness: Empirical Ethics in Care, Inaugural lecture. Amsterdam: University of Amsterdam; 2013

Section 2

# Volunteers in Palliative Care

Chapter 4

# Volunteering in Palliative Care in France: "A Tough Job"; Patient, Family, Caregiver, and Volunteer Perspectives

Yaël Tibi-Lévy and Martine Bungener

Additional information is available at the end of the chapter

http://dx.doi.org/10.5772/intechopen.69754

**Abstract**

This chapter discusses the place of volunteering in palliative care in the context of hospital services in France, and the meaning each actor gives to that presence. Its aim is to go beyond general normative discourse on the role of these volunteers in order to highlight their actions from a little-explored perspective (awkwardness, fears, reticence their activity can create) but one essential to their development. We attempt to understand how (and within what work settings) personnel and volunteers "work" together, and how that lay presence is perceived by patients and families. This research is based on a literature review and individual semi-structured interviews with patients, families, medical personnel, and volunteers in 10 hospitals. In all, 114 persons were interviewed in three work settings: palliative care units, mobile palliative care teams, and traditional services. The analysis highlighted a diversity of perceptions on volunteering, as a function of the type of actors involved and the work setting. It raises the question of the role of nonprofessional actors in hospitals, and of what form volunteering in palliative care should take in France, where volunteers explained they "are there" not "to do", but just "to be there out of human solidarity".

**Keywords:** palliative care, volunteering, qualitative research, quality improvement, models of care, France

## 1. Introduction

### 1.1. National and international context

As defined by the World Health Organization (WHO), "palliative care is an approach that improves the quality of life of patients and their families facing the problems associated with life-threatening illness, through the prevention and relief of suffering by means of early identification and impeccable assessment and treatment of pain and other problems, physical, psychosocial, and spiritual". Originating in the United Kingdom and Canada in the 1960s, this care model is based on a multidisciplinary approach, bringing together professionals and volunteers, with a shared view of improving the quality of care and strengthening social relationships. It consists in both alleviating the symptoms from which these people may suffer and putting an end to the image of place of death (often associated with death in institutions) by getting people from civil society involved in the care facilities [1]. While professionals essentially carry out care, hotel, and administrative functions within a salaried and skilled work environment, volunteers offer their time, away from their own family and theoretically through pure "altruism", expecting nothing in return [2]. This is a "free and gratuitous gesture" which "is opposed to the present society founded on wages and profit," and which some authors consider "a higher form of solidarity" [3].

Given its profoundly humanist nature, this care model has expanded rapidly throughout the world. In 2000, there were already 87 countries that have set up palliative care programs, 2/3 of them being middle or low-income countries [4]. Palliative care is found today on the five continents in forms more or less faithful to the original model and varying as a function of national policies, health systems, cultural differences, and local needs [5–7]. According to WHO, there are today 20 million people a year who require palliative care throughout the world (of whom nearly 70% are adults over 60 years) [6]. France has not escaped this phenomenon of acculturation to palliative care; the first palliative care unit (PCU) was opened in 1987—30 years ago [8]. Since the law of June 9, 1999, palliative care is considered a right "for every citizen that needs it" and a public health priority. The first national development plan for palliative care that followed (1999–2001) took the first steps in offering care, which today has become quite significant and diversified, even though the notion of "hospice," dear to the English and Canadians, was not used to bring about this development,[1] with rare exceptions (such as the *Maison Médicale Jeanne Garnier* in Paris, which has 81 beds, all devoted to caring for people needing palliative care). According to recent statistics, in 2016, France had 143 PCUs, 406 palliative care support teams (PCSTs), 5057 "identified palliative care beds" (that is, beds in curative care services, but reserved for patients needing palliative care), 92 home care organizations, 11 coordinated networks, 15 regional pediatric teams, and 350 associations of volunteers [9]. These associations place their activities within a framework of non-abandonment and nonmarginalization of people confronted with a serious illness, old age, death, and grief [10]. In this context, volunteers—estimated at 6000 persons—have the goal of "improving the living conditions of persons who suffer, in a spirit of partnership with health professionals" [11] and of "participating in changing perceptions" concerning death and severe illness [12].

[1]Indeed, France chose an original path compared to the pioneering countries: develop palliative care, not in large institutions devoted exclusively to this care, but rather in all facilities where these patients may be found. After having put in place PCUs and mobile teams for 15 years, present efforts are thus aimed at raising awareness for the "palliative approach" among all caregivers caring for people at the end of life, regardless of where they work [13–15].

### 1.2. Major issues involved in volunteering in palliative care

Although ministerial and association texts encourage caregiving teams to have recourse to volunteers, national and international literature shows that there is a certain contradiction between the attention they are regularly given and the mistrust their presence sometimes provokes in the field [16]. As Godbout emphasizes, "the idea of giving one's time [to strangers] troubles the modern mind [and often seems] suspicious" in our production-driven societies [3]. Being neither caregivers, family members nor paid workers, volunteers raise questions on more than one level for the other actors, as does the public health researcher, anxious to better understand care practices and to analyze their principal stakes.

#### *1.2.1. Giving/receiving: a delicate balance*

There is a good deal of research on the motivations of volunteers in palliative care [2, 17–24]. These works show that while volunteers are inspired in the first place by a desire to help others and therefore by altruistic and philanthropic values, they are often interested in seeking benefits for themselves as well, with these two types of motivation becoming interwoven, evolving over time and varying according to countries' cultures. Their desire to "give" is often linked (but not always) to the death in a hospice of one of their own family members: future volunteers thus wish to offer to others the quality of care received at that time. "Giving up my time is the least I can do" argues some volunteers. At other times, their system of values and beliefs motivates them to become volunteers, without them necessarily having suffered a loss: it is important for them to ensure that patients do not die alone, to lessen their suffering as much as possible, and to show them warmth and compassion through human solidarity. On other occasion, it is simply a chance discovery of palliative care that leads them to become volunteers. But even if they expect nothing in return for the help, they consciously give, on the other hand, they often admit "receiving" in return sometimes more than they give; the fact of giving does not prevent one from receiving in turn, in a circular dynamic beneficial to all. They evoke their need to feel useful to society, to seek an interruption in their daily routine, to create relationships with other people with the same values as their own, or to acquire new experiences (that they can then use to enhance their professional life, for example). Consequently, some volunteers consider the time spent among people at the end of life as a "gift", even a "privilege", from which they say they gain both enrichment and satisfaction. For Claxton-Oldfield, this relationship should be strongly encouraged as it leads to a "win-win situation" [25]. Indeed, according to him: (1) thanks to volunteers, patients, and families benefit from emotional support, assistance, and companionship in what they are going through; and (2) because of their activities, volunteers experience personal growth, which enables them to choose more easily between what is important in life and what is not. Thus, Beasley concurs that their view of the world may gain in understanding, which can help them better appreciate their own existence [19]. Ferreira considers that palliative care volunteers also contribute some relief in caregivers' busy schedules, to the point of becoming "indispensable" in some places [24].

Thus, the difference between "giving" and "receiving" rests in a delicate balance. This may be a source of stress (even of guilt) for volunteers on the one hand and of unease (even mistrust) for the other actors (patients, families, and caregivers) on the other hand. This potential stress and unease are related to the fact that the primary motivation of these volunteers is not always unambiguous, and their actions are part of end-of-life situations, a fact which may be disconcerting. In this context, and despite the goodwill of all, tensions may appear, exposing volunteers to numerous emotional challenges and their associations to important training challenges. These include teaching volunteers to maintain limits with the persons visited, to manage the emotions they themselves may be feeling, to learn to offer one's presence without imposing it… These are challenges familiar to associations and necessitate frequent retraining of their teams [16]. Some authors warn volunteers (and not only palliative care volunteers) about the feeling of "negative debt", even "inferiority" that can arise among some beneficiaries (because of the impossibility of being able to repay what the volunteer has given to them) and that may increase the latter's suffering [3]. To rebalance the debt, volunteers are sometimes recommended not to hesitate to tell patients "the extent to which their accompaniment brings just as much to themselves" [16]. Although aiming to be comforting, this parenthetical remark is not without risks and may perplex some patients who are fragile and vulnerable because of what they are going through. In fact, volunteers that have been studied constantly question the nature of their commitment, which may lead them to eventually end it [24].

The ambivalence of many volunteers regarding "concern for the other" and "concern for oneself",[2] to use the expression of Papadaniel [21], is important and merits further investigations in France, as in other countries. In spite of the challenges it raises, it must be noted that this question is nearly always approached from a single perspective, that of the volunteers and their associations, thus (voluntarily or not) putting to one side the positions of other actors. In fact, the perception patients, their families, and caregivers have of volunteers—whose motivations may sometimes appear vague—remain unclear, despite its major interest. Comparing these perspectives would enable shedding light on an activity with numerous gray areas and stimulate discussion on the question of the "effectiveness" of volunteers' activities, a theme that has recently emerged in the literature because of increasing regulatory policies and the growing importance given to evidence-based medicine [2]. Thus, in spite of the difficulty of evaluating the results of volunteers' contributions to palliative care, research work is increasingly attempting to measure the impact of their presence on patients' quality of life [26–29]. Beyond the question of "giving and/or receiving," it is becoming increasingly important to evaluate the concrete contributions of these people to the quality of care of patients in advanced or terminal stages of illness, contributions that include reduction of patient isolation, more adequate consideration of their emotional needs, an increase in life expectancy, improvement in satisfaction of families, a lightening of the burden on caregivers, etc. This evaluation should be done using proven research techniques (randomization of the study population, use of standardized and validated scales, meta-analyses…). In spite of interest for evaluation studies, routine in the area of medicine and their frequent demonstration of the positive impact of the presence of volunteers, the great majority of studies consulted almost exclusively explore the point of view of volunteers, not looking at (or only indirectly) the much less well-known perspectives of the three other types of actors involved by this care: that of patients (who are at the heart of the care process and of volunteers' concerns), that of

[2]"Souci de l'autre" and "souci de soi" in the original French text [21].

their families (who entrust their dying loved ones to an institution), and that of caregivers (whether they work in palliative care). And yet, two things appear clear: these people have probably much to say about how they perceive volunteering in palliative care and the methodological and ethical difficulties in gathering this type of information (useful ultimately for improving the quality of care to be given) are perhaps not insurmountable.

*1.2.2. Complementarity/substitution: toward professionalization of volunteering*

An analysis of the national and international literature brings to light a second type of challenge for volunteering in palliative care: it concerns the place and role of lay actors in hospital departments and the ever-present risk of the substitution of caregivers by volunteers. As Watts emphasizes for the United Kingdom, for example, the years 1980–1990 were marked by a certain professionalization of the volunteer sector in England, following encouragement by successive governments for a more active civil society [2]. In fact, hospices today have "a significant volunteer workforce to help with the care of patients and their families both in the setting of the hospice and in the community" [2, 30], and this increase in unpaid volunteer work resulted in a decrease in the growth of employment in the field [2]. These volunteers ensure a diversity of functions (from welcoming patients and families to grief support and including chauffeuring, reflexology or shop keeping). They are required to take intensive training and go through trial periods beforehand, which give them an increasingly semi-professional role [2]. Like caregivers, they must also ensure the continuity of care and their mission by following high standards of quality. Their work is becoming less and less flexible (for example, for going on vacation or in choosing the department to which they wish to offer their services), and their activity henceforth resembles "paid work, but without the pay" [2]. In addition, the original model of English hospices is increasingly contested [2], and today takes various forms, depending on the regions of the world and the needs of the populations [6]. The differences compared to the original model are especially noticeable in low-income countries, where volunteers—who work primarily in the home within the framework of community programs—may be required to give nutritional advice to patients they see [31] or may receive payment for the time spent on their visit [2]. The absence of a clear line between volunteers and professionals is fully justified in this case by the political, financial, health, and cultural context, which is very different from that in the United Kingdom but is neither wished for nor advisable in other care contexts. We will come back to this below.

The risk of volunteering veering from complementarity toward substitution is very much present in Quebec as well, where volunteer associations are increasingly preoccupied by the difficulty of defining clear boundaries for volunteer action while remaining flexible [16]. Some volunteers have a sanctioned role there, which sometimes creates dissension between volunteers looking for rewarding work and salaried personnel, who are called upon to delegate thankless tasks to them (such as folding laundry, disinfecting toys, or straightening up certain rooms) [32]. Even though it appears delicate to transform relationships that give meaning to life into tasks, the need for a clearer identification of these actions has gradually been imposed on certain association leaders, who are anxious to collaborate effectively with caregivers while staying in a role that is in their own area of responsibility [16, 33]. After having carried out an applied research project on the question, a group of Quebec researchers recently compiled a list of tasks or roles that volunteers can assume [16, 33]. These tasks or roles distinguish on one hand, those that fall into the category of instrumental acts (shop for patients, offer coffee to their relatives, describe the services offered by their associations…), and on the other, those that belong to social relationships (ensure a presence with the patient, listen to them, be attentive to their family members…). Some negotiation is always possible depending on the patient's and family members' needs for accompaniment. Volunteers should thus always demonstrate pragmatism by adapting on a case-by-case basis, while avoiding encroaching on the work of the caregivers. For them, "Doing" is often a pretext for establishing a relationship with patients and their families and enables them to more easily carry out their work of accompaniment, which is based on "Being"[3] [16]. Therefore, there is always the fear among association heads in Quebec that volunteering—given the growing shortage of resources in health care facilities and the ever-increasing need for rationalization of hospital expenditures—becomes "instrumentalized" by health care providers and public authorities, who transform this activity based on the gift of self into a form of "work at a discount" [16]. Consequently, one of the main challenges facing Quebec is neither to seek volunteers with the aim (more or less implicit) of compensating for shortcomings in the health care system nor to use them for complex tasks generally done by paid services [16].

This increasingly frequent tendency to require professional competencies from volunteers and to drift toward unsalaried employment is not specific to the United Kingdom or to Quebec. It is mentioned for many other types of volunteering and in multiple countries, such as Switzerland, where there appears to be an ongoing standardization of the behavior and role of volunteers via a sometimes overly instrumentalized vision of their training [34]. Similarly, in Belgium, hospital volunteers may be charged with running the hospital library, managing the palliative care families' homes, organizing activities, or rendering a multiplicity of services to the caregivers (such as taking the patient to the hairdresser, buying them a newspaper, or carrying the new arrivals' baggage) [35]. While volunteers cost nothing to the institutions that recruit them and automatically increase the efficiency of the facilities where they serve, given all these risks, the boundaries between volunteering and work that should not be crossed are clearly established in France, at once by associations of volunteers, by palliative care professionals, and by policies. Within this framework, it is clearly stated that volunteers must neither take the place of caregivers nor carry out semi-professional duties but limit themselves to accompanying patients and families, who desire it, by offering their presence. Thus, the Public Health Code specifies that "volunteers, trained in end-of-life accompaniment and belonging to associations that have selected them, with the consent of the patient or his or her family and without interfering with the practice of medical and paramedical care, may provide support to the care team by participating in the final accompaniment of the patient and by bringing comfort to the psychological and social environment of the patient and his or her family". In the same spirit, the circular of March 25, 2008, defines the role of volunteers in French palliative care as follows "to propose a presence, an attentiveness, discreetly and with respect for otherness, nonjudgmentally and with respect for the privacy of the sick person and his/her family life [and], on behalf of society, demonstrate kindness to those who are suffering, thereby reinforcing a sense of their belonging to the human community." This model, based purely on

[3]We will discuss this point in more detail (Section 3.2).

"Being" as opposed to "Doing", is therefore far removed from the English or Quebec models in particular and raises many questions that are rarely or never explored today: how do volunteers experience the missions entrusted to them on a daily basis? What do the caregivers say about this offer of time, which is complementary to their own? How do patients and families talk about the volunteer presence in hospital services and do they take advantage of it?

### 1.3. Study objectives

Volunteers are largely present in PCUs—where they share the same values as the caregivers in respecting the comfort and dignity of people at the end of life [36]—and to a lesser degree, in traditional hospital services. However, the way they perceive their own activity and are viewed by other actors is rarely addressed in France in official texts (from ministries or associations) or in publications. While some research has looked at volunteering in general [37, 38], other work has been focused totally [21] or partially [1] on volunteer activity as death approaches, and solely from the perspective of volunteers, who are often reticent in discussing the difficulties they encounter in carrying out their missions. Even though international publications in the past 5 years have reported a number of investigations on the volunteer experience in palliative care [2, 17–20, 22, 23], two important questions remain insufficiently studied: (1) that of obstacles and conflicts volunteers may encounter during their activity [39–41]; (2) that of the perception that patients, families, and caregivers have of this type of volunteering, whose main challenges we have described above. At most, some authors arrive at the notion of a game where all the actors are winners, with each one gaining a substantial benefit from volunteer activities [24, 25], and where volunteers say they are satisfied with their activity (in spite of the tensions noted) [24, 39, 41].

In a profoundly changing environment concerning death and the dissemination of palliative care throughout the world, the objective of this chapter is to examine the place and role of palliative care volunteers in French hospitals, in order to enrich existing analyses and provide a forum for dialog with countries where the same issues can arise. These include the following: what meaning does each person (and not only volunteers) give to this time spent in proximity to death? How, why, and within what framework do health personnel and volunteers work together? How is this unusual presence interpreted by patients and their families, that is, by those persons for whom these activities are primarily intended? Our aim is therefore to emphasize volunteers' activities from a little-explored perspective but one essential to their accomplishment—the awkwardness, fears, and reticence their activities can provoke. This entails both highlighting the way each person talks about this activity (with what terminology, what assessments, and what line of reasoning) as well as identifying any friction or dissension. This will enable redefining what is at stake and thus contribute to better care for persons at the end of their life, as well as better support for their relatives. This examination is all the more justified in light of the different volunteer experiences taking place in other countries concerning this activity [6, 42, 43] and in other health care settings in France [44]. Moreover, these examples give rise to lively and more general debate regarding the presence of lay actors in health care facilities, especially in curative services with a high degree of technicity, where the organization of work at the approach of death differs from that of the PCUs and where suspicions held by caregivers concerning volunteers are usually strong [45, 46].

### 1.4. Methodology: qualitative research among a diversity of actors in palliative care

In an attempt to go beyond broad normative discourse on the role of volunteering in palliative care, and the research that often dwells exclusively on the perspective of volunteers, we have drawn on a body of individual semi-structured interviews carried out in 10 hospitals with volunteers, but also with medical personnel (working in palliative care or not), with patients and families. The hospitals have varied characteristics in terms of location and status (Paris/Province, public/private hospitals, hospitals of varying size, and cancer centers). They all had a PCU or a PCST. They were chosen randomly from a list drawn up by the French Society of Accompaniment and Palliative Care (SFAP) of all palliative care teams in France. This methodological choice to diversify the settings was based on the hypothesis that the volunteer work under examination would be associated with a plurality of perceptions, related to both the types of actors interviewed (volunteers, caregivers, patients, families) and to the specificities of the workplace (PCU, PCST, or traditional service).

In all, five PCUs, five PCSTs, and 15 curative care services working with a PCST were investigated using interviews carried out by an experienced sociologist. The general topic emphasized was that of improving the quality of care in the facilities and meeting the needs and expectations of hospitalized people and their families. After obtaining required consent and ensuring anonymity for participants and teams studied, contact was made with the heads of different teams, with an aim for a diversity of situations. The material collected is composed of 114 interviews: 25 with patients hospitalized in PCUs, 25 with one of their family members (usually the spouse of the patient interviewed), 56 with caregivers (physicians, nurses, nurses' aides, psychologists), and eight with volunteers with good knowledge and experience of this practice (most of them were also responsible for running their association). It should be noted here that, out of the 10 palliative care teams studied, two worked without recourse to a volunteer team, which reduced our sample of volunteers to eight instead of 10. However, this enriched the analysis on the absence of volunteers in some PCUs or PCSTs and on the reasons for this absence.

All of these people were recruited using a purposeful sampling technique adapted to the type of service studied. (1) In PCUs, the four types of actors were interviewed for each site: an experienced volunteer, caregivers (either freely willing or proposed by the head of the team), patients, and families (those present the day of the study, physically and psychologically able to participate in the interview and having given their consent at least the day before to participate, after receiving detailed information on the objective of the research, their right to withdraw and the informal nature of the interviews); (2) In PCSTs, the recruitment procedure was different in two respects: since these were small teams, it was sometimes possible to interview all the personnel; as these were teams that visited traditional services solely on a request to help them out [47], neither patients nor families could be interviewed; (3) In curative care services, the recruitment of caregivers was done in two stages: an initial request made of the PCSTs interviewed to introduce us to three curative care services in their hospital, followed by a request for interviews made to the care supervisor of each of these services. As in the case of the PCSTs, it was not possible to meet patients and families here, with some patients not even aware they were in a palliative stage.

The interviews (face-to-face and recorded) were all fully transcribed and then analyzed using a grid created *a posteriori* using an inductive approach. While our initial research question broadly addressed the work of palliative care teams [48], we observed a high degree of diversity in comments made by different persons concerning volunteering, which led us to consider *a posteriori* this activity as an important dimension for an understanding of palliative care. We, therefore, extracted all references to volunteer service from the general body of interviews to study them separately using content analysis, that is, by the systematic and methodical examination of each interview. It is this analysis that we wish to present here. In order to have sufficient contextual elements and material for discussion, we have also carried out a review of the literature on volunteering in palliative care in France and in the rest of the world. This bibliographic research was done largely at the Documentation Service of the Centre National de Ressources "Soins Palliatifs" (CNDR).[4] Only the most relevant articles were used to write this chapter, which does not pretend to be exhaustive but rather to suggest several further directions of enquiry.

## 2. Results: divided opinions concerning a complex and controversial presence

In describing these results,[5] we will give priority to a presentation by type of actor, first hearing from volunteers, then from those who are at the center of their attention and of professional care (the patients and their families, who give contrasting assessments of this type of volunteering) and finally from health personnel (with often divided opinions depending on whether they work in the area of palliative care). Beyond strong differences in points of view on volunteering in palliative care (notably as a function of the status of the person interviewed and the work setting), the data bring to light several controversial issues that are largely unrecognized and concern the place and role of these nonprofessional actors among hospitalized patients receiving palliative care.

### 2.1. The viewpoint of volunteers: "being there to be there"

What do volunteers queried about their palliative care activities say and how do they adapt to the realities of the care setting? According to the general description given by a PCST caregiver whom we also interviewed, it's "a tough job" because of the strict guidelines related to this commitment and the concrete conditions for putting them into practice.

[4]This service, located in Paris, has a database of 20,000 references on palliative care, the end of life and death (the database palli@doc, accessible on line via the site VigiPallia). This database is composed of documents from journals, books, university research, conference proceedings, but also articles found in non "palliative care" journals, obtained either through document tracking or by regular communication with the BDSP (a French document network of information on public health).

[5]Most of the results in this chapter were presented in an article in French [49].

### 2.1.1. *An ambiguous commitment*

The heterogeneity in terms of age, place of activities, status, and motivations of the volunteers we met contrasts with the homogeneity of their narratives. Indeed, they described the palliative care model and their missions in quite similar terms: "*represent civil society to show these people that we are not abandoning them*", "*ensure a presence and a willingness to listen*", "*make oneself useful*", "*do things in a humane way for the person*", and "*be there to be there*". Their statements followed associative charters and current texts (that use the terms "*assistance*", "*giving*" and "*human solidarity*"), which suggests they had internalized the objectives firmly anchored in the "Being" of their association. Similarly, the rules governing this volunteering were directly quoted ("*always knock on the door before entering the room*", "*never sit down without being asked to*", "*respect the confidentiality of what is heard*"…), as were the techniques to be used (the more or less spontaneous "*hallway encounters*", "*tissues always ready in one's pocket*" or "*the coffee ploy*" that consists of offering some to people in order "*to more easily create a relationship with them*").

These standardized narratives, unassumingly expressed at times ("*We don't contribute much*"), mentioned the challenges to be met such as the initial and continuing training of these volunteers, the fact they are not substitutes for caregivers (following the principle of "*complementarity*") or the "*proper distance*" to be maintained with the other actors. The rare differences in the narratives were related more to individual modes of functioning or the setting rather than to disagreements about their duties. Thus, while some liked to have a minimum of information before entering a room "*to know what to expect*", others preferred "*not to have any prior knowledge in order to be fresh for each contact*". While some go "*to see all the patients without exception, except those not wishing to see them*", others "*never go into a room without having received an oral transmission from the caregivers*", who function as filters and informants. While some "*always refer everything to the caregivers, if possible orally and as a precaution,*" others do not want "*to bother them unnecessarily in their work, [preferring] to leave a written record and only when it involves a change in care.*"

As altruistic as their commitment is, it is not without ambivalence, however:

> *"I am very, very happy to have made this choice, in spite of all I have done in my lifetime. I am lucky to have children, grandchildren, music, lots of things anyway. Well, this really gave a new meaning to my life".*

Conscious of this personal benefit, some felt they receive more than they give, such as this woman:

> *"We must stop portraying volunteering as this beautiful image of those who give: we simultaneously receive more than we give […]. I always tell people: wait, I came to see you, but you gave me something as well. I was very pleased to get to know you".*

This ambivalence sometimes leads them to ask themselves: "*What am I doing here?,*" "*Would this person like me to look at them in this way?,*" "*Am I just feeding the beast?*" This last formulation, tinted with "guilt", questions their role among terminally ill patients, and beyond that, the potential and involuntary nuisance created by their presence. The discrepancy between giving and receiving is sometimes so strong that some are forced to suspend their activity:

> *"It's clearly something that bothers me a great deal, this part about receiving more than I give. At one time, I even stopped for six months because I felt that it was totally inappropriate of me to feed on that, while they are the ones suffering from an illness".*

One volunteer concluded that what is important is to *"not use that to feel better oneself"* and to continually question one's motivations.

*2.1.2. More or less complicated relationships with health personnel*

Working as a volunteer with palliative care professionals entails building relationships, from simple juxtapositions between the care team and volunteers to true collaboration, depending on what roles the latter are given. In some PCUs, volunteers move around according to requests from personnel, after having been introduced to patients. They play a welcoming and monitoring role and are invited to staff meetings to share their knowledge and are offered training and support sessions. Whether relationships are close or distant, all those interviewed nevertheless repeated the leitmotif that *"they are there to be there"*, *"to listen"* and have a *"common commitment"* with caregivers, not as a substitute for them but to assist them. Some then adopted a clear-cut position between what is their responsibility (*"welcome people at admissions, ensure a presence with solitary patients, give support to families…"*) and what is not (*"make beds, put patients into armchairs, give them bedpans…"*). When patient or family requests are considered outside their responsibility, they tell them they *"don't know how to or cannot"* respond; they then relay the request to the appropriate person. This position of intermediary is also adopted according to how they feel about a situation: for example, when they see particular suffering in a patient, notice unusual behavior of a relative or observe a family with a problem needing to be solved.

The relationships volunteers have with caregivers in curative care departments are more complex than with teams in palliative care and also involve an initial task of persuasion. The narratives reveal two patterns depending on the practices of the department in collaborating with volunteer associations: (1) In the first pattern, volunteers consider themselves well integrated with relatively easy access to rooms, since their role is defined and legitimated by the departmental project. The PCST indicates what patients are to be visited (after informing patients and caregivers concerned), then volunteers go to them after having received some information and checked by the nursing station. Sometimes, caregivers in these departments indicate patients directly to them, independently of the PCST, but volunteers say that in these cases, they have little information available, not even knowing if the PCST has already been by. (2) In the second pattern, access of volunteers to rooms is described as difficult. The *"first reaction"* of caregivers is one of incomprehension (*"Don't go in there; he is at the end of life"*). *"Not being able to impose their participation"* (even when there was a prior contract with the department or even if they were sent by the PCST) generates a feeling of *"transparency"*[6] and of *"frustration"*. Regretting that too few patients benefit from their presence, they confided that they sometimes take (*"a step to one side* [in relation to their code of ethics] *for the good of all"*) by going into some rooms anyway using certain tricks (by *"using relationships already established in the departments"* or by *"sneaking around"*). In the face of this resistance by caregivers—which gives them the *"impression of walking on eggshells"* and echoes later statements by some caregivers—they blame external factors such as the *"apprehension"* the caregivers have of them, the compartmentalization of departments or even the strategy of certain units *"to avoid asking for outside help in order to defend their jobs in a difficult financial context"*, thus begging

[6]A feeling of being invisible and useless.

the question of whether caregivers may simply be motivated to protect patients. To overcome this resistance, they work to make themselves better known by the departments, through awareness campaigns on volunteering, for example. In this framework, some volunteers confided in their inability to get the PCST to intercede on behalf of patients that they think are in need, with mobile teams meeting the same resistance. They then underlined the influence of departmental heads and nurse supervisors in properly integrating both the PCSTs and themselves, that is to say, integrating external actors.

### *2.1.3. Occasionally awkward situations with patients and families*

The desire of volunteers to give patients and their families *"a space for expressing themselves"* is based on the assumption they *"need compassion"* and that listening to them can *"do them a world of good"*. Although apparently simple, this position exposes them to awkward situations, sown with paradoxical injunctions, and requires them to constantly watch what they say. Thus, if they introduce themselves at the outset as volunteers, they must also be vigilant to *"never pronounce the name of [their] association"* (which may *"hurt, chock and inhibit people"*). While they are alert to *"the slightest desires"* of patients, they avoid *"questioning them"* about things considered sensitive (their family situation, their religious beliefs...). If they wish to give them their support, they are also careful to *"remain discreet"* even when patients and families use them as *"buffers"* or *"ventilate"* with regard to caregivers. They can, however, fluctuate between intrusiveness and avoidance in three cases: (1) when a patient confesses to not taking medication and they hesitate between respecting this "secret" and passing it on to caregivers; (2) when a family refuses to let volunteers visit their family member, which sometimes leads them to meet that family to explain their approach; (3) when they ensure a "silent presence" beside the patient in a coma and their mission consists precisely in doing nothing. The following excerpt illustrates the tensions they experience at these times:

> *"I had a very difficult accompaniment [...]. It was a man I had already accompanied, and he was in a coma. [...] I placed a finger on his arm and said to him: 'you see, don't be afraid, it's me, it's FIRST NAME, a volunteer, I'm going to spend some time with you.' I reassured and calmed him. [...] I stayed a very long time next to him. I knew he was very much alone, that he was afraid to die, he had said so. And so I said to myself, 'I'm going to stay next to him'. But staying silent and respectful for more than 20 minutes is very difficult because you can't think about your evening dinner. Because thoughts wander about. So at most, you can look at the painting in the room... but not look to see what the weather is like outside. I have to look at the person to really stay with him. [...] And if you look at him, you're obliged to notice certain things, but I tell myself: 'I'm being impolite. Would he like for me to look at him so that I see the inside of his mouth, would this man like that?' [...] And after a time, I tell myself: 'It would be better if I left, because I don't think I'm being appropriate.'"*

Faced with these dilemmas, some volunteers emphasized the necessity of knowing how *"to protect oneself"* by avoiding becoming *"too attached to people [or] personally investing too much"*, and they reformulated various facets of their "guilt": being *"powerless"* to relieve some kinds of suffering, involuntarily lacking respect for patients, learning about a death immediately after having left a room, or receiving more than giving. Nevertheless, these considerations do not call into question the content of their missions, which remain strongly in the "Being".

http://dx.doi.org/10.5772/intechopen.69754

### 2.1.4. *A significant marshaling of resources*

If a volunteer dismisses the idea of evaluating her presence through a tautology ("*One shouldn't think about that, but act as a volunteer should. What use is it to know that 90% of people are highly satisfied?*"), others say on the contrary, "*they always have [this question] on their minds*". They then marshal institutional and personal resources in order to improve their performance.

Institutional resources enable training for accompaniment and reduce deviant behaviors through a rigorous selection of candidates, the obligation to belong to an association, to take occasionally intensive training, and to attend regular meetings supervised by coordinators. "*It's a real uphill battle to become a volunteer and to stay one*!" noted one of them. Some training courses (on how to listen or to manage stress in particular) were described as valuable resources. They take the form of "*simulations*", "*role playing*", or of "*mimes*". They teach them to "*reformulate what people say by acting as their mirror*" and "*to not haul out their own emotions, which would be visible and prevent them being totally present with the person they are with, for the time they are there*". While the objective is to protect caregivers, patients, and families from inappropriate attitudes while shielding volunteers from overinvesting, the result is visible in the homogeneity of the narratives recorded and their correspondence with transmitted norms, without reference to their margin of autonomy.

Personal resources are intellectual and emotional in nature. According to some, they become intertwined and refined with "*experience*". Even if "*situations frequently speak for themselves*" ("*often eloquent*" expressions), "*tools*" help the volunteers adjust the content of their presence: these include the "*observation*" of peoples' behavior when the volunteers arrive, the "*interpretation*" of the signals sent, the "*intuition*" of what should be done or said, their "*feeling*" about the quality of encounters, in a word, "*perceptiveness*" or "*listening to oneself*". The principle is always the same: "*conduct yourself according to the persons and the situations*", while bearing in mind how "*to define oneself as an accompanying volunteer*". One person explained that this implies "*being clear about oneself and one's own past*". Some help themselves by taking personal "notes" after each encounter to use as a reminder and to provide guidance concerning the proper attitude to take both with regard to patients and to themselves. Others rely on subtle signs: a patient who "*says it was nice of them to come*", a family that "*demonstrates friendliness*", and caregivers who say they "*are pleased with what the volunteers contribute*". One interviewee thus felt that "*feedback from caregivers [is] a more reliable indicator*" for judging the soundness of their activities than expressions by patients and families since it was a reflection of the quality of "*collaborative partnerships*" with caregivers, and "*it's not just because a patient was aggressive that a visit was not important*". In doing this, she shifts the purpose of volunteer activity toward the caregivers (what is important is that the departments are satisfied).

## 2.2. The viewpoint of patients and families: a very clear-cut narrative

In contrast to the rather formal and uniform narratives of volunteers, comments by patients and families proved pragmatic and diversified, ranging from praise to disapproval, together with indifference and mistrust. Four groups with differing opinions, independent of the age or sex of the interviewees, stand out: positive, distant, mistrustful, and hostile.

### 2.2.1. *"Volunteers: charming and devoted people"*

A first group of patients and families emphasized, sometimes strongly, the relationship qualities of volunteers encountered in the PCU. While the word "kindness" is often mentioned, many terms also evoked volunteers' positive attitudes (*"friendly, charming, likeable, smiling, present, helpful, devoted, considerate, good listeners, discreet, reassuring, big hearted, marvelous, fantastic"*). Some patients said they appreciated the fact volunteers came by to say hello with *"a handshake"*, allowing them *"to chat,"* and sometimes took them on a tour of the hospital grounds. *"It's a plus here, because I saw the sun again, I once more saw several people from outside, and I appreciated that"* (a patient). These narratives highlight the importance to some patients of being listened to and respected, needs that are often mentioned by volunteers and palliative care professionals. For their part, families welcomed the *"idea [of volunteers] devoting some time to others"*, considering that *"their approach [is or must be] beneficial"* at several levels. For example, they enable patients to *"talk about things they like"* and to *"feel free"*; give them *"a helping hand"* such as dialing a telephone number; run the family day room of the PCU and give out coffee there; furnish information; or *serve as intermediaries* with caregivers in order *"not to unnecessarily divert the personnel"* from their work, added the father of a patient.

Whether they come from patients or from relatives acting as spokesperson and protector for their ill family member, these narratives reveal two styles of expression, sometimes based on personal experience, sometimes on abstract considerations. The former referred to concrete experiences. *"We talk with the volunteers about anything that exists in order to think of other things a little, and it feels good"*, and it positively underlined volunteers' commitment:

> *"They devote themselves to us until 6 pm… Sometimes, I feel bad about that, and I say to myself 'oh my, those poor people'." (a patient).*

> *"They very kindly visited Mama, but they saw she was very well looked after. So, taking the burden off volunteers is also a good idea." (daughter of a patient).*

Some families pointed out the *"reassuring"* side of this presence, which does what they themselves cannot do: ensure a permanent presence next to their relatives be a rampart against the harshness of hospital life. This was expressed by three women:

> *"Volunteers reassure me because I know that my husband is not alone and these are people from outside the medical milieu, they are people like you and me".*

> *"With them, I can leave with peace of mind, knowing that my son will not be abandoned".*

> *"Once, a lady came, my husband was asleep, and I wanted to make a telephone call, but I didn't dare leave him alone. She offered to stay with him while I was gone. And it worked out very well. He didn't realize it, and I was free from anxiety".*

These narratives based on experience reflect a contrasting attitude to the mistrust families have concerning the hospital system, felt to be dehumanizing. This suggests that the need for a presence next to patients, often mentioned by volunteers and partisans of palliative care, originates as well in a need expressed by families worried about their ill relative.

The second narrative style is based on hypothetical scenarios—*"I think that if I can't walk anymore, I'll ask volunteers to buy my morning newspaper"*—or on impersonal considerations—*"It's *valuable to have someone who can give you a hand"*. This wording borrows much from comments described above and from those of certain caregivers, since they refer to the dominant ideas about volunteering, testifying to the permeability of representations on the subject. It also points out the variety of "little favors" that volunteers can render in addition to their mission of listening and being present, and the more general functions such as their role of third party or informant. People using this style nevertheless proved not to be very talkative about any personal experiences: "*Yes, I met the volunteers, yes, yes, always lots of commitment*". And some comments were ambiguous: "*They're not really disagreeable*", "*I'm not lucky because each time they come, I have people here or I sleep some*". This vagueness suggests that some people accept a volunteer's visit, not because they wish to, but because they do not dare refuse or criticize it.

### 2.2.2. *"It's for isolated people or for afterwards!"*

A second group of patients or families adhered to the same narrative concerning volunteers but distanced it from their own experiences. While recognizing volunteers' potential value, they insisted on the fact their presence is "*mainly helpful to others*" (those who have few visits) but not to themselves:

> *"For patients whose family lives far away or is absent or non-existent, I think that it can definitely be positive; for now, I am happy to have exchanged a few words with people who go by, but…" (a patient).*

> *"Volunteers are very helpful in other people's rooms, because you have people here who don't have any family…" (the daughter of a patient).*

These narratives, usually succinct as concerns volunteering, show on the one hand that some people do not have a need themselves for this presence, which they do not wish to experience, and on the other hand that, according to them, volunteering activity should be first directed toward isolated patients. Some reserved the possibility of changing their opinion depending on the evolution of their situation, and put off that opportunity for later. "*Perhaps someday I'd be very happy to see volunteer…*", one patient hinted.

### 2.2.3. *A position of "mistrust"*

A third group was indifferent to, mistrusted, or was even embarrassed by the presence of volunteers. Not inclined to meet them, three patients spoke in unequivocal terms:

> *"It doesn't upset me that they come by to see me, but it wouldn't bother me if there weren't any, you see; I don't really want to talk".*

> *"Personally, that doesn't interest me much. The person comes in at any time of the day, and you have to initiate a topic and then keep up the conversation… It's not my thing".*

> *"I don't think I need volunteers. First, because I have difficulty speaking so I don't want to talk. And then, what is it I have to listen to? Their personal history. It's not worth it".*

Their reticence is associated with discomfort, something rarely mentioned by volunteers interviewed, even though some caregivers allude to it. This is discomfort at having to accept that people who are not part of the personnel come into their room, often without warning, having to spend time with these people who "*have doubtless personally experienced the death of a family member"*, having to talk with them, even when they do not wish to or have the ability to do so... Volunteers' motivations seem to them *a priori* suspicious, which concurs with the opinions of some of the caregivers in curative care facilities. They even speculated about the impetus behind the volunteer commitment and the safeguards to be put in place, like this patient who worried "*that volunteers commit some faux pas*" that can be harmful to patients, and he raised the question of their supervision: "*I don't know how it happens [he said] but with some... It could have the opposite effect of what is intended, for sure*".

Some families took a similar position. Emphasizing that volunteers should not impose their presence on untalkative patients, they identified with their relatives:

> *"I'm a little like my mother, I don't really want to talk... I don't really like to describe my life... and besides, it's so personal and so difficult, what we're going through now, that we don't necessarily want to open up to strangers."*

Families then put forward their knowledge of their family member's character ("*My father really doesn't want to see volunteers, he's very unsociable and doesn't like to be bothered or have someone come and ask him questions*") or of their preference for getting by without help ("*My mother is someone who has always taken care of herself. So, I don't think she wants to see volunteers*"). For these families, as spokespersons for their relatives, this volunteer presence is secondary, because the essential in their eyes is clinical in nature: "*What's important in a hospital, it's doctors, nurses. Then, the rest...*" (daughter of a patient). A wife stood out here by justifying her mistrust through fear that volunteers prove to be too talkative, due to the fact they have doubtless suffered grief:

> *"I don't know if volunteers are like that, but people who have lost a loved one, often tell you too many things. Me, I'm not ready to open the doors. There are things I don't want to know, so...."*

#### 2.2.4. *"A fairly revolting presence"*

Finally, a few persons were conspicuous by their caustic remarks, considering this presence as "*fairly revolting*". For one patient, it is "*the black mark, the big problem*" because of their "*systematic infantilizing and disagreeable body language of pity*", their "*manner of more or less forcing themselves into the rooms*" and their "*way of putting patients in a position of inferiority*". She described her impressions at length:

> *"They're sort of into 'oh, my poor lady, how are you?' [...] They touch you without asking whether you want to be touched. [...] I've even had some take my foot, like for a child, and try to tickle me. [...] The problem is that I left my door open because I'm claustrophobic, so they took that as an invitation. When they came in and I didn't want it, I would say to them: 'what can I do for you?'. It was a sort of joke that should have made them understand I was not interested. And some answered: 'OK, it's you who wants to do something for us?' So, they practically forced me into the position of being sick, of being the poor person that must be helped at all costs".*

According to her, they are pursuing "a kind of dangerous quest for good deed, that is harmful and nonconstructive", which brings her to question the attitude of "Being" without "Doing":

> *"What good is it to visit someone who didn't ask for it, bringing your pity with you, when the person doesn't need it? Volunteering is not a state, but a dynamic process: they need to come with an active approach, like the clowns who go see the children to amuse them, for example. They need to come with*

*a project and concrete proposals such as activities or some entertainment for example, but not wander from room to room, hoping that at the right moment, the person will want to have their hand patted or be served a cup of coffee".*

This rejection of the essence of volunteering based on the gift of presence (*"being there to be there"*) is here aligned with a strongly rejected notion of "pity". It is prompted by a lack of "dynamics" where volunteers apparently make a choice beforehand of a territory and mode of intervention. This last excerpt in particular identifies the unintentional annoyance that volunteering can carry with it in palliative care in France. Beyond considerations of the best position to adopt as an accompanying volunteer of the end of life (give/receive, complementarity/substitution), it is the question of what content to give to volunteering between "Being" and "Doing" that is at issue here, and with it, one part of the model of French palliative care. We will discuss this at greater length (see Section 3.2.2).

### 2.3. The viewpoint of health personnel: contrasting opinions

Narratives recorded among caregivers in palliative care (PCU or PCST) and in curative services are characterized by profound differences depending on the professional setting of those that express them and their concept of end of life care. Indeed, the former, coming from a palliative care milieu, favor volunteering for the most part, while the latter, from outside, are more distant.

#### 2.3.1. *Often-convinced palliative care professionals*

The perspective of palliative care professionals on volunteers was predominately favorable, especially in PCUs where a positive, even indispensable, place is accorded to them from the outset. The help volunteers provide them, especially if there is a lack of personnel, was thus evoked with qualifiers such as *"full members"* of the team, *"intermediaries"* between patients and caregivers, or *"valuable assistants"* in multiple domains. These include greeting and installing patients in their room, offering a presence and an ear to isolated patients, watching over agitated persons, responding *"to people's need for conversation"*, *"being there"* symbolically during dying and transfer of the body, participating in religious rites (if the family asks for this), accompanying mourners to the funeral parlor, ensuring follow-up of grieving (in sup port groups led jointly by psychologists or in the home), or managing *"solidarity funds"*. Their ability to communicate important information to teams was also underlined: observing that *"families talk more freely to volunteers than to themselves"* (because of their *"friendly, attentive and available"* qualities, and the absence of "a white coat" one caregiver adds), some teams invite them to their unit meetings to give their perspective and help them *"refocus"* follow-up care. Sometimes the transmission notebook used for communication between volunteers may be consulted by the caregivers, referral contacts are assigned to them, they are given specific training (in addition to that of their association), and occasional or regular meetings are organized between caregivers and volunteers. While this organization of collective care activity accords volunteers a special place and is a reflection of their positive integration in the units, it raises the question of the blurred and shifting boundary between work and volunteering, mentioned in the case of other countries (see Section 1.2.2).

Contrary to caregivers working in PCUs, those in PCSTs do not have their own space for carrying out their activity. Indeed, they move about, following requests from curative services to provide their skills and are thus subject to the rules in these services, including those concerning recourse to volunteer work. This makes their working conditions insecure and uncertain. Some interviewees regretted that this work organization limits a volunteer presence considered useful for some patients. One caregiver described the effects of a lack of workspace for her PCST, limiting opportunities to meet volunteers: *"We would like to work more with volunteers, but where could we locate a volunteer center when already the psychologists don't have a place for seeing a patient that isn't hospitalized?"* While they share the same model as their PCU colleagues, PCST caregivers have to adjust to a work setting that is less receptive and that requires them to be accepted there before negotiating a place for volunteers. The latter would often be *"unwelcome"* in the units, even if they *"try to introduce themselves to explain what they do"* and even when the PCST considers their visit would help certain patients. *"The real problem is that, in the hospital, everyone defends his or her territory, and you'd better not tread on it"* [said a PCST caregiver]. In the departmentalized context of typical services, according to this person, volunteers are seen as trespassers, who are all the less legitimate to intervene because they are at once nonprofessionals, outside the medical milieu, and concerned with the end of life. Therefore, PCST personnel must be vigilant in their use of volunteers to avoid a situation where their own services may no longer be requested by certain caregivers.

### *2.3.2. The rare but critical discourse of palliative care physicians*

Unfavorable remarks on volunteering, and thus less expected, were voiced by two physicians rather reluctant to support the place of volunteers in the palliative approach. One was a supervisor of a PCU and one a supervisor of a PCST. Critical of current practices in palliative care, their reflections launched a heated debate and echoed to negative remarks made by certain patients and families.

While the first denounced an *"over-accompaniment"* of patients in PCUs and voiced doubts as to the place to be accorded volunteers, the second *"wondered"* about all forms of volunteering from the moment they are practiced in a hospital. According to him, too many people already gravitate around the patient, it is not proper that *"non caregivers know things about patients, sometimes without their knowledge" and "even if people are free to refuse to see them, they don't always do so for fear of the consequences"*. The volunteers' motivations also seemed ambiguous to him: *"I even seem to have seen some volunteers who came here because they also felt the need to talk to someone"*. He, therefore, said he was *"skeptical as to the respect for professional confidentiality, to which they are theoretically bound"*, *"conflicted"* as to *"the place they should be given,"* and finally, *"reticent"* to collaborate with them in his PCST, *"except for people who have no family members"*. Noting that some curative care services had *"walls"* that were difficult to get past for people outside the service (volunteers or members of mobile teams), he has decided to let volunteers *"manage by themselves"* in getting in and accessing rooms, solving the problem of the double constraint mentioned earlier.

> *"I told volunteers: I can't get into that, you have to go see the supervisors or the physicians, discuss what you do, the agreement made with the hospital, your limits, confidentiality, and see if they agree that you can intervene."*

#### 2.3.3. *Often-mistrustful caregivers in curative care services*

While caregivers from PCUs and PCSTs described numerous details of their relationship with volunteers, those from curative care departments often had little to say on the subject. This was perhaps due to shorter interviews because of a lack of personnel (the interview then concentrated on their work with patients at the end of life); it was because they said they already had all the necessary resources: "*We have the PCST and a psychologist in the service*" or because they did not know "*how things worked with volunteers*"; or it was because, as a matter of principle, they did not think volunteers had a place among patients in a palliative stage, and they thus avoided directing them to the patients. "*I often hesitate to do it [...]. So if they really want to go there, they go. But I tell them, because I don't think they necessarily have the training for it. It's delicate...*" (a nurse supervisor). The reticence of caregivers can doubtless also be partly explained by the very medicalized, hierarchical, and bureaucratic functioning of many services, where the professional aspect dominates the nonprofessional, and the technical aspect takes precedence over the relational.

Only one caregiver stated, briefly but explicitly, that the presence of volunteers was "*a plus*" for the patients and for their families. Her position of openness breaks with the caricatural image that opposes a curative care milieu—rebelling against accompanying volunteers—to one favorable to palliative care and thus paves the way for genuine collaboration in acute care units.

## 3. Discussion: redefine the stakes of volunteering in palliative care in France

Two central themes for discussion can be highlighted. The first examines the weak overlapping of comments, representations, and experiences reported by the different actors we interviewed: these differences in discourse relate both to work settings that are more or less favorable to this type of voluntary service and to more or less high expectations concerning volunteers. The second theme concerns perspectives for the development of volunteering in palliative care in France and reexamines the concept of "being there".

### 3.1. Expectations and work settings more or less suitable for volunteer service

The narratives studied show that there are strong differences in the perception—and therefore in the acceptance—of the presence of volunteers, depending on whether the caregivers work in a palliative or in curative care setting. This is a reflection of two dominant and opposing conceptions of care: one palliative, endowed primarily with human resources and centered on relieving symptoms; the other curative, sometimes very technical and focused on cure [48]. In the first case, volunteers are often considered full members of the care team; in the second case, they are sometimes mistrusted by caregivers, even though the two positions—somewhat overstated here—need to be tempered depending on the sites and people interviewed, as we noted above.

### *3.1.1. Palliative care volunteers in PCUs*

There are numerous similarities between France and the countries described above in Section 1.2 of this chapter concerning the meaning volunteers give to their action and the place assigned to them by PCUs. According to statements shared by volunteers and the majority of palliative care professionals interviewed, offering one's time is synonymous with "citizen commitment well beyond the world of health", as noted by R. Aubry, coordinator of the national Program for the development of palliative care 2008–2012 at the Ministry of Health and President of the End-of-Life Observatory [50]. According to the narrative common to most of the volunteers and caregivers interviewed, the time that is offered enables giving support to patients (even if the curative treatments have become ineffective) and brings a "breath of fresh air from the outside", to use the expression of Ferreira [24]. Because of the common values held by the people interviewed, collaboration between caregivers and volunteers is satisfying in most cases. But as the sociologist M. Castra has noted, good integration of volunteers into palliative care facilities may also be explained by the fact that "the PCU personnel quickly understood the advantages to be had by a volunteer presence for their own work comfort", especially at times of heightened activity [1]. Henceforth, and even if volunteering is by definition an unpaid activity, it can sometimes resemble work—for free—resembling in several ways the professional world. This is translated concretely into an expansion of the division of work in peripheral activities, with the more or less formal delegation of caregivers' relationship tasks to volunteers (settling incoming patients into their rooms, informing, being a presence, attentive listening, watching over agitated patients…). In this context, some interviews suggested the idea of a relative professionalization of volunteering in palliative care, an idea all the more compelling in that several interviewees underscored the criteria for selection, training, and strict monitoring (even quasi managerial) that govern them. These elements carry the risk of a political instrumentalization of volunteering in order to make up for the financial shortfalls of care facilities and to thus attempt to compensate for the crisis of the Welfare State. This is reminiscent of fears expressed by association leaders in other countries [16]; that of the potential breakdown of the boundaries between employment and volunteering, fears that in fact exist in a diversity of contexts other than that of palliative care and health [37].

If the risk of boundaries breaking down exists, it should nevertheless be put into perspective by the uniqueness of the object of this accompaniment—the end of life—but also by all the preventive measures taken by French volunteer associations to restrict the activity of their teams as much as possible to the strict accompaniment of patients and their family (listening, presence, limited small favors). Consequently, the people interviewed rejected the idea of work on the cheap as much as that of the professionalization of their activity. They considered that this political and "too categorical" way of reasoning "confined them to techniques that create barriers" between them and those they come to help, and they then evoked a basic principle—that of their complementarity with the caregivers. They also rejected the idea of an instrumentalization of their action by care facilities in order to reduce costs. They justified the many rules to which they are subjected by citing the concern of the associations to train them to adopt the proper attitudes and to "protect" them from risks of overinvestment. These rules—from the world of salaried employment—thus appear to be mainly "safeguards" destined on the one hand to select "people with sufficient moral qualities" to visit patients at the end of life, and on the other, to "integrate this lay work into a hospital setting", itself highly regulated and hierarchical, as noted by some French authors [1, 43]. The transfer of skills to volunteers would therefore reflect more a "rite of institutionalization" than a professionalization, which again, is not specific to the volunteering we studied, but to all volunteering, from the moment, there is a close relationship between volunteers and those they help [37].

Beyond these considerations, the literature shows that being a volunteer in a PCU or in a hospice is not devoid of stressors, which pose important training challenges to volunteer associations, notably in teaching how to manage one's emotions. Sources of stress may include occasionally ambiguous roles in relation to caregivers and other personnel, unclear status, at times difficult relationships with patients, families, or caregivers, personal problems that can sometimes disrupt the life of volunteers… [39]. Several volunteers in our study thus mentioned several sources of stress: the guilt they felt from time to time at the idea of receiving from patients more than they give them; their regular questioning of their commitment and of their true motivations; their efforts to not deviate from a "position of listening and being present" to one of doing tasks that would be the responsibility of professionals; the awkward situations they can find themselves in (such as a silent presence at the side of someone in a coma); and the whole battery of institutional and personal resources they constantly mobilize. In fact, some palliative care teams today have difficulty in retaining their volunteers [2], and France is no exception. Even though this topic was not addressed as such in our interviews and would thus merit further investigation, it does indeed emerge implicitly in some narratives, such as that of the woman who, although highly dedicated, admitted having suspended her volunteer activities for 6 months because she felt so uncomfortable in certain situations. To limit pressures, some authors emphasize the importance on the one hand of avoiding "unrealistic expectations" that may come from caregivers, patients, or families (through better information on staying within the limits) [16], and on the other hand, the need to reward volunteers more for the social bond they try to re-establish between the patient and society, following the example of what is observed in the world of work [2, 51–54]. Nevertheless, it has been observed that all the volunteers interviewed spoke with enthusiasm about their work alongside caregivers, a result found in other studies, and that some authors explain by the strategies that volunteers use more or less consciously in adapting to stressing situations [39, 41]. According to some research, these coping strategies, in association with proper supervision of volunteers by their association, diminish their feeling of burn out and malaise, to the point they do not always view their activities as stressful in spite of the various tensions identified [39, 40]. It thus appears that the goodwill with which the volunteers studied fulfill as best they can the missions given them constitutes in itself an important resource for the PCUs as well as for hospices, as Watts also observes for the United Kingdom [2].

### 3.1.2. *Palliative care volunteers in PCSTs and in traditional care facilities*

As we noted in the introduction (see Section 1.1), France made the original choice of developing institutionalized palliative care, not in large facilities dedicated solely to people needing this care, but directly in hospital departments, where the vast majority of deaths occur.

This was done initially and over a period of 15 years by the creation of palliative care teams (PCUs and PCSTs), considered as expert at improving end-of-life conditions in the hospital. In a second phase since 2004, the "palliative culture" was disseminated among all hospital caregivers frequently faced with the death of their patients [13–15]. Compared with the original model for hospices and what can be observed in many countries, this new direction can be explained by both the concern of French policies to ensure that patients could be cared for in the facility where they were usually hospitalized—and thus by the same caregivers as those that had taken care of them since their first symptoms—and by the critical necessity of rationalizing expenses.

Although the issue of integrating volunteers into PCUs and hospices is well documented, there is still little data on the participation of these lay actors in acute care services, as some authors have recently emphasized [55, 56]. In this respect, this research provides some information, at least for France. First, while these volunteers used the same terms as those attached to a PCU in talking about their commitment and their missions[7] (attesting to a close proximity between them), on the other hand, they described their access to patient rooms as much more difficult in curative care facilities than in PCUs. This is similar to other research. Thus, a study carried out among Jalmalv[8] associations shows that their volunteers "are not yet quite at home in the place they are committed to", and that their action resembles more a "juxtaposition of teams" than a "true collaboration" with unit caregivers [45], because of "misunderstandings and presuppositions" (more than from "frank opposition") [43]. In curative facilities, these situations revive unresolved tensions concerning the proper moment to change from curative to palliative care [57]. This requires volunteers to work in an uncertain environment and constantly exposes them to feelings of invisibility, of uselessness and frustration, also observed by Finkel [58]. According to some, these difficulties can be explained by a "poor understanding in the facilities of [not only] the notion of palliative care, [but also] of the indispensable help given by volunteers" [43], bearing in mind—as other authors note—that "it takes very little to call into question the [always fragile] cohabitation between caregivers and volunteers" [59]. Some associations attempt to get past this resistance by organizing campaigns to raise awareness of volunteering in order to become better known to caregivers in their hospital [60] and by working to set up "partnership collaborations" with traditional departments [61]. They thus have to think ahead of time about "the optimal placement" of their teams [43] and then actively defend their position, as emphasized by Delaloye in the context of Swiss hospitals as well [56]. However, this is not specific to volunteering in palliative care. The functions of caregiver and volunteer (regardless of what they are) "are in fact sources of misunderstanding [and] conflicts" for several reasons: misunderstanding of volunteering on the part of care professionals, competition around care activities, frequent lack of recognition of each one's role, the infrequency of shared projects, and the ever-increasing turnover in personnel [46]. Some authors also mention the risk of a lack of continuity of volunteer presence in acute care services, and the necessity for their associations to "invent new functions", even if it is necessary to "reassess our goals" [46]. Conversely, some volunteers, better integrated into the

[7]Listening to and giving support to patients and their families, human solidarity, the gift of presence…

[8]Jalmalv ("Jusqu'à la mort, accompagner la vie", "Until death, accompany life"): one of the main French associations of palliative care volunteers.

facilities, mention with regret their inability to get the PCST involved with patients who they think are in need, as these cross-disciplinary teams encounter the same obstacles to intervening as they themselves do [48].

Although work conditions for volunteers in traditional care units are more difficult than in PCUs, the volunteers interviewed were, however, less pessimistic than these authors on the development of their activity. They reported largely satisfactory conditions of collaboration with some acute care units that were more aware of and open to palliative care and volunteering than others were. Some interviewees thus emphasized the influence of heads of departments and supervisory nurses in their proper integration, with the mobilization of all personnel proving to be essential as well, as also stated by Verchère [62]. French publications describe other successful experiments at integrating volunteers outside of PCUs [63–65]. These experiments are doubtless destined to multiply the given political will to disseminate the palliative culture in all facilities that are frequently confronted with the death of their patients. According to Bird—who is interested in volunteer accompaniment in English acute care hospitals—volunteers trained in palliative care, through their careful listening and support, make a substantial contribution alongside caregivers in better responding to the needs of people at the end of life and their families: "when medicine can do no more, a smile, a touch and a friend are the best prescription—this is what our volunteers have in abundance", she argues [55]. She emphasizes that training programs set up for that purpose are necessary but not sufficient. To be effective, they should be accompanied by both regular support from recruited volunteers and communication activities to make them better known by facilities that are potentially interested. Another direction mentioned simultaneously by American [66] and Canadian [67] authors consists in raising the awareness of future physicians about issues linked to the end of life by proposing they spend several hours as a volunteer in a hospice during their first year of study. This work shows that the students who followed these programs—pilot programs for now—acquired very positive experience for themselves and for their future profession, whether in reducing fear in the face of death, in encouraging their personal reflections, or in learning to better communicate with patients and families.

### 3.2. Between "Being" and "Doing": should volunteer service in palliative care be re-examined?

The above results lead us to a reexamination of the place and role—between "Being" and "Doing"—of volunteers in French palliative care and to suggest some avenues of reflection in order to strengthen its development and ensure its sustainability.

#### *3.2.1. "Being there"*

The comparison of narratives between volunteers, caregivers, patients, and families in France shows the extent to which volunteering in palliative care is conceptually integrated into "Being", as the President of Jalmalv also points out [10]. Presence and listening are at the heart of the system, with a clear emphasis on not substituting for caregivers and of discretion concerning patients and their families. As in the Swiss model, volunteers in French palliative care say they are engaged in a relationship with the other, based on not abandoning vulnerable people and on a civil society determined to care for its members [34]. These social skills ("*savoir-être*"), sometimes referred to as an "art" due to the multiple "adjustments" involved [68] are appreciated by some patients and families interviewed and by most palliative care professionals, especially when there is a need to go to the bedside of isolated people or play a welcoming or monitoring role. These results reinforce what is already known, as well as the fact that volunteers studied gain benefits from their ethical commitment [1, 12, 21]. But they also reveal several new elements: the intentional absence of volunteers in two palliative care teams interviewed, which is contrary to the prevailing view that "a care facility cannot be palliative if it has not integrated volunteers into its multidisciplinary team" [12]; the reluctance of some caregivers in curative facilities to co-operate with them as a matter of precaution; the numerous efforts of the associations to make their missions known to the acute care staff and thus, to gain access to the rooms of more patients; a mixed or even hostile perception by certain patients and families of this type of volunteering; or the discomfort, often kept quiet, of some volunteers in certain situations (guilt in receiving more than they give, difficult presence with some patients in a coma, use of tricks to access certain rooms in curative care facilities …).

The concept of "being there", used by many voluntary associations, is a central notion in several countries, a "precious thing" which consists of "creating value through encounters" [69]. This concept is especially appropriate for French palliative care volunteers, whose recurring position, strongly voiced by their associations, is "to be there" just "to be there" through solidarity. This relationship skill, which rests primarily on presence and active listening, is an integral part of the basic training for people wishing to become volunteers in palliative care, and of continuing education for those who already are. As emphasized by the French association "Accompaniment in Palliative Care" (ASP) in its training pamphlets, "listening is the tool par excellence of the volunteer". It is what enables them to be truly there, for the time they are there, with the person for whom they are there, and is what shapes them. However, if "learning to listen" is a major challenge for a good accompanying volunteer, other aptitudes are also needed. In France, as elsewhere, these volunteers must therefore participate in several other forms of training in order to fulfill and experience their missions to the fullest. For example, they must learn to manage their emotions—become "hardened" regardless of the empathy they may feel for some patients—and to not go beyond the limits of activity set by their associations [2]. Some studies also note that one of the important challenges faced by these social skills today is to improve taking cultural differences into account, due to the considerable diversification of the patient population in hospices and PCUs[9] [2, 70, 71]. Indeed, these studies find gaps concerning cultural competencies among volunteers in place and thus an urgent need for remediation. In particular, it is necessary for these actors to learn to "be there" for all people, regardless of their ethnic origin, language, religion, or beliefs, and to offer each one, without discrimination, an appropriate accompaniment. According to Jovanovic, improving this type of skill is "vital, crucial, and imperative" in reducing the social exclusion of some patients [70]. She, therefore, makes several recommendations to achieve this, such as online access for volunteers to certain downloadable documentary resources or the creation of an interactive web site [71]. Although these publications concern the United Kingdom (Watts)

[9]Depending on the country: Muslims, Asians, Africans Hindus, Filipinos, East Europeans…

and Canada (Jovanovic), they can be completely superimposed on the French situation, where the same problems are to be found or soon will be, in a context where social skills are greatly needed.

*3.2.2. "Doing": a pretext for "Being". Toward a more active volunteering in palliative care?*

The position of French volunteers in palliative care, exclusively in the "Being" camp rather than the "Doing" camp, constitutes a source of "pride" for some association leaders [10]. However, it may also constitute a significant obstacle to the development of this activity in France, given the resistance to making a place for volunteers expressed by some health personnel, patients and families in our study. Indeed, in spite of strong institutional recognition, these types of voluntary associations paradoxically suffer today from a "structural fragility". There are "a limited number" of contracts in the field, recruitment as well as fidelity of their members is becoming problematic, the integration of volunteers into facilities is proving "laborious," and volunteering appears to be "disappearing from the preoccupations" of palliative care teams themselves [10], a problem calling for urgent reflection. Our review of the literature shows in particular that there is one important difference between France and most of the other countries studied. In France, palliative care volunteers focus on attentive listening, support and little favors (thus reducing their role strictly to "accompaniment"), whereas elsewhere, "accompanying volunteers" are, but a small group among all active palliative care volunteers. The latter carry out a multitude of quasi-professional tasks (receptionists, secretaries, drivers; reflexologists, fundraisers…), as we have seen in Section 1.2.2 [2, 16, 32, 42, 43]. They can be present with hospitalized patients, as well as with those in day care or in home care, sometimes even offering their professional skills in a wide range of activities (supplementary therapists, hairdressers, spiritual care workers, qualified nurses, doctors…) [72]. In some places, their contribution may be especially beneficial to patients, families, and caregivers alike. This is notably the case in the United Kingdom in pediatric palliative care facilities, where volunteers provide a number of different services, such as organizing recreational activities for hospitalized children and their siblings, playing the role of schoolteachers, providing supplementary therapies, giving support to parents, and managing the families' homes [73]. As emphasized by Sévigny for Quebec [16] and Gérardy for Belgium [35], the "Doing" of volunteers (and not only those in palliative care) is often a pretext for "Being", an excuse to more easily initiate contact with patients and families. More than the task or small favor ("Doing"), what is important above all is the creation of relationships ("Being"). "Doing" provides the possibility to create relationships that would otherwise never have existed to generate an atmosphere of confidence and to keep an expert eye on changes in behavior in case they need communicating to caregivers. In this sense, "Doing" is not necessarily the goal to attain, but the means chosen to better give support to those that need it through the presence being offered.

By improving care without raising costs, this type of action doubtless has a strong development potential for volunteering in palliative care, and can be transferred—at least in theory—to France. Indeed, the literature review and the interviews carried out reveal several avenues for the growth of volunteering in French palliative care. Examples would be of volunteers entering patients' rooms with "concrete proposals" (loaning books or CDs, distributing snacks at various times of the day, doing small errands, organizing entertainment, helping patients move around inside and/or outside the hospital…). That would give them pretexts considered by some interviewees as more "acceptable" than just "*wandering from room to room, hoping that at the right moment, the person will want to have their hand patted or be served a cup of coffee*" (quoting the disapproving comments of one of the patients encountered). But in return, this implies an extension of their activity to include "service", similar to what is observed in other countries studied. French experiments are moving toward more active volunteering, such as at *La Maison de Gardanne*, where volunteers are asked (in addition to just being present) to help patients with their breakfast, to go from room to room proposing menus, to help the cooks, or to organize outings [63]. However, such an expansion offends both political (health authorities) and ideological (volunteer associations) sensibilities surrounding the central principle of strict complementarity between professionals and volunteers and creates the risk—considered omnipresent—of seeing this type of volunteering turned into a form of work on the cheap. This probably explains why none of the volunteers interviewed mentioned the idea of expanding their mission to include more concrete activities, thus in a way concealing tensions in the workplace and shunning the potential opportunities mentioned above. We should note here that the restriction in France of volunteer action to a presence and attentive listening constitutes a unique feature of volunteering in palliative care. In other care settings, "Doing" is indeed considered as important as "Being", in the name of the usefulness and effectiveness of volunteer involvement. This is particularly the case for associations to fight cancer, where volunteers are responsible for doing prevention, collecting funds, or helping to personally redeploy patients [44].

## 4. Conclusion

While volunteers have a strong presence next to palliative care professionals, their activity remains poorly understood, notably in France. This chapter draws on a literature review and interviews with volunteers, caregivers, patients, and families. It discusses the place and role of these actors and examines their perspectives for development in the French context. Premised on generosity, volunteering is, in fact, a complex activity, sometimes controversial, and often described as a "tough job". On the one hand, it is clear that the apparent conceptual consensus disseminated by the model of palliative care concerning the beneficial presence of volunteers among hospitalized patients at the end of life becomes fragmented in the field into a wide diversity of perceptions (related to the status of the actors involved, to their concept of care as death approaches, and, where appropriate, to their work setting). On the other hand, it appears that the dominant concept among volunteers interviewed, "being there to be there", leads to poorly recognized tensions, but which are capable of compromising the sustainability of volunteering and its development in curative care facilities. This raises the question of frameworks and resources needed to overcome resistance and to facilitate the desired dissemination of the "palliative culture" among all health workers confronted with the end of life [13–15]. More broadly, this study shows that the sometimes difficult acceptability of hospital volunteers (and not only those in palliative care) by those persons they wish to help without a prior request (in this case, patients hospitalized in palliative care) depends in part on the fact that, in France, care is and remains for many people "the exclusive domain of salaried health personnel" [74] (even within the specific framework of palliative care units or teams). This suggests that attitudes change more slowly than policies on this question.

In addition, this analysis highlights similarities and differences between volunteering in palliative care in France and in several other countries. These differences, more or less marked, are due to both palliative care policies carried out in these various countries and to cultural elements that are more or less favorable to the presence of lay actors at the side of caregivers. Depending on the country, this presence may manifest itself in a nearly exclusive attitude of listening and kindness (as in France) or as a semi-professional position where volunteers are responsible for carrying out a multitude of tasks (as in the United States, Canada, and the United Kingdom). While these two positions are justifiable, they give a considerable stimulus to discussion and reflection and suggest directions for fruitful research projects. Beyond the debate on the risk of instrumentalizing volunteering in order to reduce costs, and on the need for better defining the boundary between work and volunteering, we should not forget that concerns are finally always and everywhere the same: improve the care of people at the end of life and their families, for a society each one hopes to make better.

## Acknowledgements

We would like to thank those in charge of the hospitals in which this study was carried out, as well as the volunteers, caregivers, patients, and families who accepted to give us some of their time, the *French National Authority for Health* for its financial support, Sylvie Amsellem for carrying out the interviews, Janine Barbot (sociologist) for her critical view, and Jon Cook for translating this text into English. We express also particular thanks to the Documentation Service of the *Centre National de Ressources "Soin Palliatif"* (CNDR) (Paris) for its substantial bibliographical contribution and particularly to Marina Renesson, Sophie Ferron, and Caroline Tête for their kindness and professionalism.

## Author details

Yaël Tibi-Lévy* and Martine Bungener

*Address all correspondence to: yael.levy@cnrs.fr

National Centre for Scientific Research (CNRS), Villejuif, France

## References

[1] Castra M. Bien mourir - Sociologie des soins palliatifs. Paris: Presses Universitaires de France, Le Lien social; 2003. 384 p

[2] Watts J. The place of volunteering in palliative care, In: Chang E and Jonhson A, editors. Contemporary and Innovative Practice in Palliative Care. Publisher InTech, 2012, 302 p, [Internet]; Available from: http://www.intechopen.com/books/contemporary-and-innovative-practice-in-palliative-care/the-place-ofvolunteering-inpalliative-care

[3] Godbout J. Bénévolat en soins palliatifs et esprit du don. In: Sévigny A, Champagne M, Guirguis-Younger M, editors. Le bénévolat en soins palliatifs ou l'art d'accompagner. Québec: Presses de l'Université Laval; 2013. pp. 15-27

[4] Jackson A. Histoire et rayonnement mondial [des soins palliatifs]. In: Jacquemin D, editors. Manuel de Soins Palliatifs. 2nd ed. Paris: Dunod; 2011. pp. 21-31

[5] Woitha K, Hasselaar J, van Beek K, Radbruch L, Jaspers B, Engels Y, Vissers K. Volunteers in palliative care—A comparison of seven European countries: A descriptive study. Pain Practice. 2015;**15**(6):572-579. DOI: 10.1111/papr.12209

[6] WHO (World Health Organization), WPCA (Worldwide Palliative Care Alliance). Global Atlas of palliative care at the end of life [Internet]. 2014. Available from: http://www.who.int/nmh/Global_Atlas_of_Palliative_Care.pdf [Accessed: 10-05-2017]

[7] Van Beek K, Woitha K, Ahmed N, Menten J, Jaspers B, Engels Y, Ahmedzai SH, Vissers K, Hasselaar J. Comparison of legislation, regulations and national health strategies for palliative care in seven European countries (Results from the Europall Research Group): A descriptive study. BMC Health Services Research. 2013;**13**:275. DOI: 10.1186/1472-6963-13-275

[8] Delbecque H. Le développement des soins palliatifs en France. In: Jacquemin D, editors. Manuel de Soins Palliatifs. 2nd ed. Paris: Dunod; 2011. pp. 28-50

[9] SFAP (Société Française d'Accompagnement et de Soins Palliatifs). Les soins palliatifs en France en quelques chiffres [Internet]. 2016. Available from: http://www.sfap.org/RUBRIQUE/EN-QUELQUES-CHIFFRES [Accessed: 10-05-2017]

[10] Le Lann P. Les associations d'accompagnement en France: enjeux et perspectives. In: Sévigny A, Champagne M, Guirguis-Younger M, editors. Le bénévolat en soins palliatifs ou l'art d'accompagner. Québec: Presses de l'Université Laval; 2013. pp. 153-176

[11] Ministère de la Santé. Circulaire n°99 du 25 mars 2008 relative à l'organisation des soins palliatifs, Définition, missions et obligations du bénévolat d'accompagnement en matière de soins palliatifs [Internet]. 2008. Available from: http://social-sante.gouv.fr/fichiers/bo/2008/08-04/ste_20080004_0100_0113.pdf [Accessed: 10-05-2017]

[12] Wagner JP. Place des bénévoles dans les unités de soins palliatifs. Pourquoi? Pour qui? Pour quoi? Pour quand?. Gerontologie et Societe. 2004;**108**:159-165

[13] Tibi-Lévy Y. La démarche palliative - Bilan à 10 ans. Médecine Palliative. 2016;**15**(4):62-68. DOI: 10.1016/j.medpal.2015.11.005

[14] Mino JC, Fournier E. Les mots des derniers soins - La démarche palliative dans la médecine contemporaine. Paris: Les Belles Lettres, Coll. Médecine & Sciences Humaines; 2008. 354 p

[15] Ministère de la Santé. Guide de bonnes pratiques d'une démarche palliative en établissements [Internet]. 2004. Available from: http://www.sfap.org/system/files/guide_bonnes_pratiques_soins_pal_ministere.pdf [Accessed: 10-05-2017]

[16] Sévigny A. L'action des bénévoles dans les soins palliatifs - Remarques à partir de l'expérience Québécoise. Sciences Sociales et Santé. 2017;**35**(2):33-41. DOI: 10.1684/sss.20170202

[17] Stelzer EM, Lang FR. Motivations of German hospice volunteers: How do they compare to nonhospice volunteers and US hospice volunteers? The American Journal of Hospice & Palliative Care. 2016;**33**(2):154-163. DOI: 10.1177/1049909114559067

[18] Nissim R, Emmerson D, O'Neill B, Marchington K, Draper H, Rodin G. Motivations, satisfaction, and fears of death and dying in residential hospice volunteers: A prospective longitudinal study. The American Journal of Hospice & Palliative Care. 2016;**33**(4):335-339. DOI: 10.1177/1049909114559830

[19] Beasley E, Brooker J, Warren N, Fletcher J, Boyle C, Ventura A, Burney S. The lived experience of volunteering in a palliative care biography service, Palliative & Supportive Care. 2015;**13**(5):1417-1425. DOI: 10.1017/S1478951515000152

[20] Garbay M, Gay MC, Claxton-Oldfield S. Motivations, death anxiety, and empathy in hospice volunteers in France, The American Journal of Hospice & Palliative Care. 2015;**32**(5):521-527. DOI: 10.1177/1049909114536978

[21] Papadaniel Y. La mort à côté. Toulouse: Anacharsis Editions, Collection Les ethnographiques; 2013. 208 p

[22] Claxton-Oldfield S, Claxton-Oldfield J, Paulovic S, Wasylkiw L. A study of the motivations of British hospice volunteers. The American Journal of Hospice & Palliative Care. 2013;**30**(6):579-586. DOI: 10.1177/1049909112462057

[23] Elliott G, Umeh K. Psychological issues in voluntary hospice care. British Journal of Nursing. 2013;**22**(7):377-383. DOI: 10.12968/bjon.2013.22.7.377

[24] Ferreira S. Quand "être avec" remplace "faire avec". Krankenpflege. Soins Infirmiers. 2013;**106**(6):68 70

[25] Claxton-Oldfield S. Hospice palliative care volunteers: The benefits for patients, family caregivers, and the volunteers. Palliative & Supportive Care. 2015;**13**(3):809-813. DOI: 10.1017/S1478951514000674

[26] Walshe C, Algorta GP, Dodd S, Hill M, Ockenden N, Payne S, Preston N. Protocol for the End-of-Life Social Action Study (ELSA): A randomised wait-list controlled trial and embedded qualitative case study evaluation assessing the causal impact of social action befriending services on end of life experience. BMC Palliative Care. 2016;**15**:60. DOI: 10.1186/s12904-016-0134-3

[27] Sallnow L, Richardson H, Murray SA, Kellehear A. The impact of a new public health approach to end-of-life care: A systematic review. Palliative Medicine. 2016;**30**(3):200-211. DOI: 10.1177/0269216315599869

[28] Horey D, Street AF, O'Connor M, Peters L, Lee SF. Training and supportive programs for palliative care volunteers in community settings. The Cochrane Database of Systematic Reviews. 2015;**7**. DOI: 10.1002/14651858.CD009500.pub2

[29] Pesut B, Hooper B, Lehbauer S, Dalhuisen M. Promoting volunteer capacity in hospice palliative care: A narrative review. The American Journal of Hospice & Palliative Care. 2014;**31**(1):69-78. DOI: 10.1177/1049909112470485

[30] Armstrong-Coster A. Living and Dying with Cancer. Cambridge: Cambridge University Press, 2004. 210 p

[31] Defellippi K, Mnguni M. Volunteers working in a community palliative care service. In: Scott R, Howlett D, editors, 2nd ed. Volunteers in Hospice and Palliative Care. Oxford: Oxford University Press; 2009. pp. 177-194

[32] Comeau E, de Varennes V. La gestion des équipes de bénévoles en soins palliatifs: tendances et défis. In: Sévigny A, Champagne M, Guirguis-Younger M, editors. Le bénévolat en soins palliatifs ou l'art d'accompagner. Québec: Presses de l'Université Laval; 2013. pp. 177-196

[33] Sévigny A, Guyon AC, Martin A, Frappier A. Collaborations bénévoles-professionnels en soins palliatifs—Intégration des bénévoles aux services de soins palliatifs, Région de la Capitale-Nationale. Québec: Institut sur le vieillissement et la participation sociale des aînés de l'Université Laval (IVPSA); 2016

[34] Cailler F, Delaloye S, Margot M, Nielsen I. Professionnalisation du bénévolat d'accompagnement: questions et enjeux dans la formation. In: Sévigny A, Champagne M, Guirguis-Younger M, editors. Le bénévolat en soins palliatifs ou l'art d'accompagner. Québec: Presses de l'Université Laval; 2013. pp. 219-237

[35] Gérardy J. L'accompagnement entre l'être et le faire: le volontariat en Belgique. ASP Liaisons. 2015;**50**:23-26

[36] ANAES (Agence Nationale d'Accréditation et d'Evaluation en Santé). Modalités de prise en charge de l'adulte nécessitant des soins palliatifs. Recommandations pour la pratique clinique [Internet]. 2002. Available from: http://www.has-sante.fr/portail/upload/docs/application/pdf/txt_soins_palliatifs_recommandations_finales_mise_en_ligne.pdf [Accessed: 10-05-2017]

[37] Simonet M. Le travail bénévole, Engagement citoyen ou travail gratuit?. Paris: La Dispute, Coll. "Travail et salariat"; 2010. 219 p

[38] Vermeersch S. Entre individualisation et participation: l'engagement associatif bénévole. Revue Française de Sociologie. 2004;**45**(4):681-710. DOI: 10.3917/rfs.454.0681

[39] Claxton-Oldfield S. Hospice palliative care volunteers: A review of commonly encountered stressors, how they cope with them, and implications for volunteer training/management. The American Journal of Hospice & Palliative Care. 2016;**33**(2):201-204. DOI: 10.1177/1049909115571545

[40] Phillips J, Andrews L, Hickman L. Role ambiguity, role conflict, or burnout: Are these areas of concern for Australian palliative care volunteers? Pilot study results. The American Journal of Hospice & Palliative Care. 2014;**31**(7):749-755. DOI: 10.1177/1049909113505195

[41] Dein S, Abbas SQ. The stresses of volunteering in a hospice: A qualitative study. Palliative Medicine. 2005;**19**(1):58-64. DOI: 10.1191/0269216305pm969oa

[42] Monroe B. Donner de son temps: le bénévolat à St Christopher's Hospice de Londres. Revue de la Fédération Jalmalv. 2009;**96**:15-18

[43] Reboul P. Bénévoles accompagnants et soignants: état des lieux et questions posées. Revue de la Fédération Jalmalv. 2009;**96**:7-14

[44] Pourtau L, de Oliveira JP, Ferrand-Bechman D. Les bénévoles "concernés" dans les associations de lutte contre le cancer en France—Spécificités et limites d'un engagement fondé sur le vécu et la 'dette'. Les Tribunes de la Santé. 2014;**42**:77-94

[45] Schaerer R, Reboul P. Où en sont les relations Soignants-Bénévoles en France ? L'expérience des associations Jalmalv. Revue de la Fédération Jalmalv. 2009;**96**:50-52

[46] Demoulin F. Les relations entre les bénévoles et soignants en établissement de santé. Revue de la Fédération Jalmalv. 2009;**96**:19-23

[47] Legrand E. Servir sans guérir. Médecine palliative en équipe mobile. Paris: Editions EHESS, Coll. En temps & lieux; 2012. 264 p

[48] Tibi-Lévy Y, Bungener M. Les avatars des soins palliatifs désenclavés - Enquête en USP, en EMSP et en service de soins curatifs, Médecine Palliative. 2014;**13**(2):57-67. DOI: 10.1016/j.medpal.2013.08.002

[49] Tibi-Lévy Y, Bungener M. "Etre là pour être là: discours croisés sur le bénévolat d'accompagnement". Sciences sociales et Santé. 2017;**35**(2):5-31. DOI: 10.1684/sss.20170201

[50] Aubry R. État des lieux du développement des soins palliatifs en France en 2010 - Rapport à M. le Président de la République et M. Le Premier Ministre [Internet]. 2011. Available from: http://social-sante.gouv.fr/IMG/pdf/Rapport_Etat_des_lieux_du_developpement_des_soins_palliatif s _en_France_en_2010.pdf [Accessed: 10-05-2017]

[51] Hamilton G. The support of volunteers. In: Scott R, Howlett S, editors. Volunteers in Hospice and Palliative Care: A Resource for Voluntary Services Mangers. 2nd ed. Oxford, New-York: Oxford University Press; 2009. pp. 87-91

[52] Claxton-Oldfield S, Jones R. Holding on to what you have got: Keeping hospice palliative care volunteers volunteering. The American Journal of Hospice & Palliative Care. 2013;**30**(5):467-472. DOI: 10.1177/1049909112453643

[53] Claxton-Oldfield S, Claxton-Oldfield J. Should I stay or should I go: A study of hospice palliative care volunteer satisfaction and retention. The American Journal of Hospice & Palliative Care. 2012;**29**(7):525-530. DOI: 10.1177/1049909111432622

[54] O'Brien, S, Wallace E. Volunteers working in a tertiary referral teaching hospital. In: Scott R, Howlett S, editors. Volunteers in Hospice and Palliative Care. 2nd ed. Oxford: Oxford University Press; 2009. pp. 195-210

[55] Bird S, Bruen G, Mayland C, Maden M, Gent M, Dilnot B, Raj J. Using volunteers to support end-of-life care. Nursing Times. 2016;**112**(14):12-14

[56] Delaloye S, Escher M, Luthy C, Piguet V, Dayer P, Cedraschi C. Volunteers trained in palliative care at the hospital: An original and dynamic resource. Palliative & Supportive Care. 2015;**13**(3):601-607. DOI: 10.1017/S1478951514000169

[57] Baszanger I. Entre traitement de la dernière chance et palliatif pur—Les frontières invisibles des innovations thérapeutiques. Sciences sociales et Santé. 2000;**18**(2):67-94. DOI: 10.3406/sosan.2000.1491

[58] Finkel C. Regards croisés bénévoles/soignants—Un témoignage. Revue de la Fédération Jalmalv. 2009;**96**:45-46

[59] Schwald R. Attentes des bénévoles, frustrations des bénévoles?. Revue de la Fédération Jalmalv. 2009;**96**:39-44

[60] Catant C. Le rôle des associations dans la mise en place et le suivi du bénévolat d'accompagnement. Revue de la Fédération Jalmalv. 2007;**96**:43-46

[61] Grimaud C. L'accompagnement des malades par les bénévoles des Petits-Frères des Pauvres. Revue Française des Affaires Sociales. 2002;**4**:53-62

[62] Verchère S. Le bénévolat dans une unité de soins palliatifs. Revue des Affaires Sociales. 2002;**4**:37-51

[63] Lapiana JM, Gourmand M, Genthier J, Daude M, Paquet I, Lepoutre B, Prévost S. Les bénévoles de La Maison de Gardanne. Revue de la Fédération Jalmalv. 2009;**96**:28-32

[64] Desfosses G, Thibaud S, Maigret P. Rôles et relations entre les bénévoles d'accompagnement et l'équipe soignante au sein de l'USP de l'hôpital des Diaconesses. Revue de la Fédération Jalmalv. 2009;**96**:24-27

[65] Mignot M. Jalmalv Allier: une "entente parfaite" avec l'équipe mobile ! Témoignage. Revue de la Fédération Jalmalv. 2009;**96**:47-49

[66] Mott ML, Gorawara-Bhat R, Marschke M, Levine S. Medical students as hospice volunteers: Reflections on an early experiential training program in end-of-life care education. Journal of Palliative Medicine. 2014;**17**(6):696-700. DOI: 10.1089/jpm.2013.0533

[67] Stecho W, Khalaf R, Prendergast P, Geerlinks A, Lingard L, Schulz V. Being a hospice volunteer influenced medical students' comfort with dying and death: A pilot study. Journal of Palliative Care. 2012;**28**(3):149-156

[68] Sévigny A, Champagne M, Guirguis-Younger M, editors. Le bénévolat en soins palliatifs ou l'art d'accompagner. Paris: Hermann; 2014. 358 p

[69] Goossensen A, Somsen J, Scott R, Pelttari L. Defining volunteering in hospice and palliative care in Europe: An EAPC White Paper. European Journal of Palliative Care. 2016;**23**(4):184-191

[70] Jovanovic M. Cultural competency and diversity among hospice palliative care volunteers. The American Journal of Hospice & Palliative Care. 2012;**29**(3):165-70. DOI: 10.1177/1049909111410415

[71] Jovanovic M. Improving cultural competency among hospice and palliative care volunteers recommendations for social policy. The American Journal of Hospice & Palliative Care. 2012;**29**(4):268-278. DOI: 10.1177/1049909111414863

[72] Burbeck R, Low J, Sampson EL, Bravery R, Hill M, Morris S, Ockenden N, Payne, S, Candy B. Volunteers in specialist palliative care: A survey of adult services in the United Kingdom. Journal of Palliative Medicine. 2014;**17**(5):568-574. DOI: 10.1089/jpm.2013.0157

[73] Burbeck R, Low J, Sampson EL, Scott R, Bravery R, Candy B. Volunteer activity in specialist paediatric palliative care: A national survey. BMJ Supportive & Palliative Care. 2015;**5**(3):287-293. DOI: 10.1136/bmjspcare-2012-000355

[74] Schaerer R. Éditorial. Revue de la Fédération Jalmalv. 2009;**96**:3-4

Section 3

# Special Circumstances

Chapter 5

# Palliative Care in Japan for Individuals with Amyotrophic Lateral Sclerosis

Mitsuko Ushikubo

Additional information is available at the end of the chapter

http://dx.doi.org/10.5772/intechopen.69773

**Abstract**

Palliative care has not been focused on noncancer yet. Amyotrophic lateral sclerosis (ALS) is a fatal, rapid progressive, and intractable neurodegenerative disease. Individuals with advanced ALS cannot perform activities of daily living by themselves, but their mental awareness remains clear. Individuals with ALS experience various pain soon after diagnosis, and a multidisciplinary team approach is needed because their pain can become complicated Caring for individuals with ALS needs to both start and end with palliative care in the physical, psychological, social, and spiritual aspects. The Japanese Ministry of Health, Labour and Welfare enacted the Principles of Policy for Rare and Intractable Diseases (*nanbyo*), which were the first set of such principles to be established in the world. This chapter describes the palliative care in Japan, from the perspectives of nursing and *nanbyo* measures. Also, three unique characteristics of ALS care in Japan are mentioned: the high level of disagreement between patients and family; the high rate of ventilator use compared with Western countries; and the low consumption of morphine. Healthcare practitioners need to apply the notion of the total pain to provide palliative care to individuals with ALS and acknowledge the challenges of providing timely symptomatic management.

**Keywords:** ALS, palliative care, total pain, end-of-life care, family care, home care support system

## 1. Introduction

Amyotrophic lateral sclerosis is the most common degenerative disease of the motor neuron system. This disease is also known as Lou Gehrig's disease. The symptoms and progression processes can be quite varied in different people.

### 1.1. Characteristics of amyotrophic lateral sclerosis

Amyotrophic lateral sclerosis (ALS) is a devastating, neurodegenerative, and progressive disease with no established treatment. ALS is characterized by muscle weakness and atrophy, and these affect the upper and lower limb movements, swallowing, speech, and respiratory function. However, bowel, bladder, and oculomotor function and sensation are spared. The cognitive and behavioral symptoms have also been described, although frank dementia is a rare occurrence [1]. Patients with ALS may die within 3–5 years after the onset of their first symptoms if they do not choose to live with a ventilator [1]. Bulbar onset type, increased age, and front temporal dementia (FTD) are prognostic factors for shorter survival [2]. The course of ALS is quite uncertain, and sudden death or unexpected death is often seen [3]. Therefore, healthcare providers should consider end-of-life care soon after the diagnosis [3].

### 1.2. Epidemiology of ALS in Japan

The number of those patients with ALS has increased remarkably. **Figure 1** shows the number of patients with ALS who were certified as eligible for receiving medical financial aid in Japan for the treatment of a designated rare and intractable disease, which increased from 860 individuals in 1979 to 9950 individuals in 2015 [4].

The incidence of ALS in the Japanese population is much lower than in the Caucasian populations of Europe and North America. The prevalence and incidence rates per 100,000 people

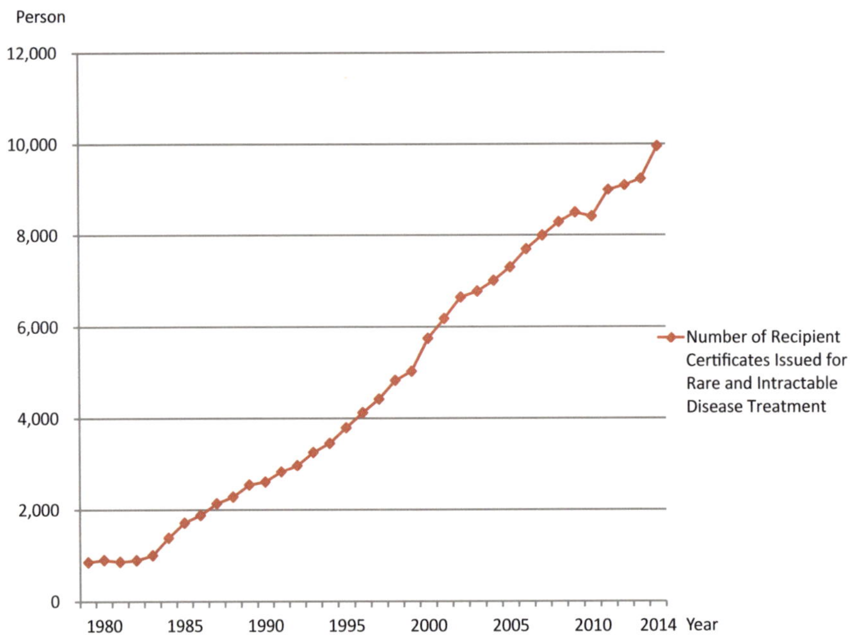


**Figure 1.** The number of ALS patients who are issued certificates in Japan for the treatment of rare and intractable disease between 1979 and 2015. Data are cited from Japan Intractable Disease Information Center [4].

per year in Japan were 9.9 and 2.2, respectively, in 2013 [5]. The highest prevalence, as well as incidence, was evident in the group comprised of individuals in their 70s, and the ratio of men to women was approximately 1.5 [5].

The aspects of ALS have also changed. A single-facility retrospective study conducted in rural Japan reported the following findings [6]. The percentage of ALS patients whose onset type was bulbar increased from 14.2% (1978–1982) to 38.3% (2008–2012) over the 35-year period of the study. The percentage of ALS patients with dementia increased from 0% (1978–1982) to 20.2% (2008–2012). The percentage of patients whose age at onset was ≥ 70 years increased from 0% (1978–1982) to 38.2% (2008–2012).

## 2. Continuous loss and decision-making accompanied by the disease progression of the disease characteristic in individuals with ALS

Individuals with ALS suffer from decreasing function in their activities of daily living (ADL), such as immobility, respiratory insufficiency, speech difficulties, and swallowing difficulties. Poor ADL performance leads to care burden. Physical pain in individuals with ALS is not proportional to the severity of the disorder [7]. Psychological distress is great even in the early stage shortly after diagnosis [8]. The reactions of the patients and their family members at the time of diagnosis need to be shared with the hospital and community care staff in order to start providing adequate support. Individuals with ALS can develop a sense of security and suppress cumulative suffering if they feel that they are supported from an early stage.

Individuals with ALS cope with relentless loss in the disease progression stage. When disease progression is fast, the patient often loses additional bodily functions before his or her illness acceptance can catch up. The patient's psychological state can be unstable due to the steady loss in physical function at a time when various difficult decisions (e.g., when and how to utilize social services and undergo medical treatment) must be made by the patient and his or her family [9].

### 2.1. Palliative care for ALS symptoms and pain

The symptomatic management should be provided in a timely manner in order to slow progression and optimize quality of life (QOL). It can be said that care for individuals with ALS starts and ends with palliative care. Symptoms of ALS which need palliative care include motor dysfunction, dyspnea, dysphagia and drooling, dysarthria, and pain. Other symptoms such as depression, anxiety, sleep disturbances, and nightmares must be addressed with specific pharmacological and no pharmacological approaches including a supportive psychotherapy, which is usually best administered as family therapy.

#### *2.1.1. Motor dysfunction and palliative care*

It causes mental distress that patients cannot perform ADL by themselves and need to be cared for by others. Individuals with ALS experience repeated falls as physical function deteriorates, which forces wheelchair dependence and eventually progresses to a bedridden condition. Living with this deterioration and disturbance in one's body image is also painful. These patients lose their jobs, and the opportunities for going out and socializing are inevitably reduced. The range of life naturally becomes narrower. Accordingly, motor dysfunction develops into a spiritual pain whereby individuals with ALS question the meaning of life, thereby exacerbating psychological and social distress [10].

Healthcare practitioners need to respect and focus on the residual abilities of the individuals with ALS—not the parts that they cannot do—and make the utmost use of what they can accomplish. It is important to find and devise a way of life with the individual with ALS and his or her family members that incorporates adequate assistive devices or utensils so that tasks can be performed by the individuals with ALS.

Although the people surrounding individuals with ALS tend to thoughtlessly reach out because of feelings of pity and kindness and prevention from danger situations, these actions can increase their mental distress of the individuals with ALS and reduce their self-esteem [10]. Technology development makes individuals with ALS do themselves by operating environmental devices, as long as they have a part of the body that they can move slightly, such as the tip of their little finger or eye tracking.

Human value is not changed at all even if the body cannot completely move. It is important for individuals with ALS to have roles and feel that he or she is needed from their surrounding friends and family. The healthcare profession needs to build up partnerships with their patients and their family members in order to enhance their autonomy and power to live.

In addition, active and passive physiotherapy has a pivotal role, especially in order to prevent muscle contractures and joint stiffness, whereas acetylcholinesterase inhibitors (e.g., pyridostigmine) may lead to a short-term improvement in muscle strength, especially during the early stages of the disease and in those with bulbar symptoms.

### *2.1.2. Respiratory dysfunction and palliative care*

If breathing cannot be adequately performed, this will directly lead to a life crisis. Patients express the respiratory disorder caused by ALS as "feeling [like I am] drowning in the sea while in the land," "feeling [like I am] being strangled with cotton," and "suffering [because I] cannot cough up phlegm." The leading cause of death of individuals with ALS is respiratory failure, and they must live with the fear of approaching death all the time.

For the early detection of respiratory disorders in homecare, healthcare practitioners need to perform peripheral oxygen saturation (SpO2) checkups during the nighttime and measure sniff nasal inspiratory pressure, the difference between chest girth at expiration and inspiration, and forced vital capacity. Symptomatic treatments such as respiratory rehabilitation, mechanical insufflation-exsufflation (MI-E), noninvasive positive pressure ventilation (NPPV), tracheostomy, and tracheostomy positive pressure ventilation (TPPV) can also be applied.

Ideally, NPPV should be introduced before the respiratory muscles are excessively exhausted. However, some patients do not undergo the early introduction of NPPV because they believe that they "do not want to live by relying on any machine" or "if [they] rely on machines, [their bodies will get] stuck." In addition, sometimes the NPPV therapy itself is only troublesome when they are not well aware of respiratory insufficiency and cannot realize the effect of NPPV.

Healthcare practitioners need to explain how symptoms can be relieved, rather than just prolong life, in order to promote a better adaptation and tolerance to NPPV. Individuals with ALS are not able to detach and attach the NPPV mask whenever they desire due to upper limb disorders. Since displacement of the mask can cause death, [3], a sufficient home care support system must be prepared for each NPPV user.

Also, a small amount of morphine provides effective relief for respiratory distress in patients with ALS [11]. Morphine consumption in Japan is lower than in other countries. According to 2008–2010 data compiled by the Ministry of Health, Labour and Welfare, morphine consumption was 204.5 g/day per 1 million persons in the United States, 191.8 g/day per 1 million persons in Canada, and only 7.2 g/day per 1 million persons in Japan [12]. The use of morphine for neurological diseases was approved by the Japanese national health insurance system in 2011 [13]. Morphine consumption can be expected to increase in the near future.

#### *2.1.3. Difficulty in swallowing and eating and palliative care*

Oral intake can become difficult as ALS progresses. Poor oral intake or dysphagia as well as difficulty with self-feeding and meal preparation leads to weight loss and malnutrition and increases the risks of aspiration pneumonia and suffocation. Moreover, poor oral intake deprives the pleasure of individuals with ALS and lowers QOL. The long time required for oral ingestion leads to fatigue. Malnutrition causes not only respiratory waste but also the loss of spirit need to think or redesign the way of future life [14].

There are many ways to increase oral intake: consider the position of the neck and head, change the patient's body posture, modify the type of food, use a thickener, conduct swallowing rehabilitation therapies, perform an esophageal laryngectomy or total laryngectomy, etc. It is also important to collaborate with professionals such as speech therapists, dentists, and certified nurses who specialize in dysphagia. Percutaneous endoscopic gastrostomy placement is also indicated.

#### *2.1.4. Difficulty in speech and palliative care*

Due to the disease progression, individuals with ALS are difficult to say what they want to say. The individuals with ALS frustrate that the things they want to convey do not pass well and experiences a sad feeling by being told that "I do not know what you are talking about" from others. Individuals with ALS may lose their voice by tracheostomy.

Communication greatly affects QOL of the individuals and their family. In recent years, remarkable progress has been made in the field of augmentative and alternative communication (AAC), which includes all forms of communication (other than oral speech) that are used to express thoughts, needs, wants, and ideas. Consequently, various communication devices and switches are available. In cooperation with speech therapists and occupational therapists, selection and contrivance of a communication device is required along with aggravation of the disease condition.

As training and time are necessary to use communication devices, it is desirable to introduce them at an early stage where the disease state is mild, but until patients do not realize the necessity, they are reluctant to introduce. It is an important key whether or not the individuals with ALS desire to convey their thoughts and whether or not their family and supporters feel like wanting to hear the individual's thoughts.

#### *2.1.5. Physical pain*

The two types of physical pain are summarized in **Table 1**. Although fasciculation—arising through degeneration of the intramuscular motor axons—and subsequent painful muscle cramps are often the first symptoms of the disease, the secondary in nature is most reported types of pain [15].

#### *2.1.6. Total pain*

As mentioned above, deterioration of physical function and various types of physical pain cause mental, social, and spiritual distress. These pains become increasingly complicated and cumulatively expand with disease progression. Therefore, the concept of "total pain" coined by

**Primary forms of pain**

- Neuropathic pain (extremities)
- Painful cramps (lower limbs, hands, abdomen)
- Spasticity (lower limbs)
- Pain caused by inability to move and change position (diffuse, including buttocks, limbs, and trunk)
- Paresis of limbs (shoulder pain, articular pain)
- Joint contractures (hand and ankle joints)
- Itch (diffuse)

**Secondary nature (most reported types of pain)**

- Neck pain due to hyposthenia of neck muscles
- Back pain due to reduced mobility
- Pressure sores due to reduced mobility
- Pain due to suctioning of phlegm
- Articular pain due to reduced mobility
- Shoulder pain due to reduced mobility
- Facial pressure ulcers due to NIV mask
- Pain due to ventilator hose pulling or weighing

**Table 1.** Types of pain in individuals with ALS, adapted from Chió et al. [15].

Dame Cicely Saunders to manage the cancer pain—which has physical, psychological, social, and spiritual components whereas the contribution of each component will be specific to each individual and his or her situation [16]—can also be applied to rare and intractable diseases [9, 13]. Pain will never be relieved by only paying attention to physical aspect (**Figure 2**). That is why individuals with ALS should be supported using a multidisciplinary team approach.

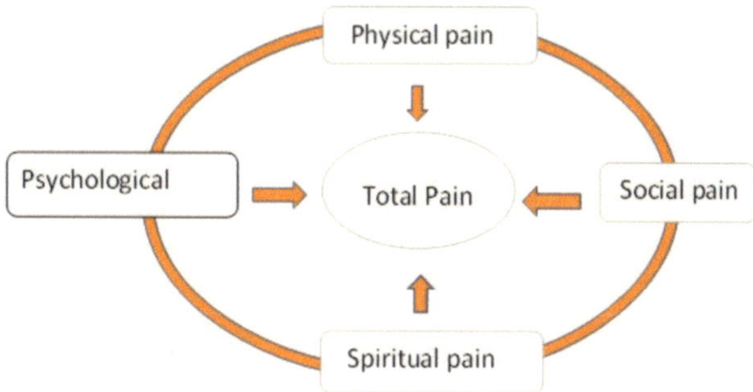


**Figure 2.** Total pain, adapted from Ushikubo [9].

## 3. Government measurements in Japan

### 3.1. Definition of "Nanbyo"

Rare and intractable diseases are called *nanbyo* in Japan. *Nanbyo* is defined by the following four conditions: (1) no known cause, (2) no clearly established treatment, (3) rare disease status, and (4) long-term care is typically required [4]. *Nanbyo* is the administrative term that the government uses to promote clinical investigations and research in order to establish effective treatments and improve cares [4]. Patients are often shocked by the poor image of the term *nanbyo*. However, they should understand the term in a positive sense. *Nanbyo* is the administrative term which has the meaning that the Japanese national government strengthens to clarify the causes of disease and effective treatments.

Patients registered as having one of the designated *Nanbyo* or the designated rare and intractable diseases are eligible to participate in a subsidy scheme that covers medical expenses. The designated *Nanbyo* selected from rare and intractable diseases that meet the following two conditions: (1) diseases with a prevalence of less than 0.1% of the population in Japan (i.e., affecting less than approximately 140,000 persons) and (2) diseases with established objective diagnostic criteria. As of April 2017, 330 rare and intractable diseases were designated [4]. The typical neuromuscular *nanbyo* includes ALS, multisystem atrophy, Parkinson's disease, spinocerebellar disease, and multiple sclerosis.

### 3.2. Historical development of Japan's governmental policy

The system of rare and intractable diseases in Japan was started ahead of the world as "*nanbyo* measures" and gradually getting improved [17]. In 1972, the Ministry of Health,

Labour and Welfare enacted the Principles of Policy for Rare and Intractable Diseases [4] which was the first set of principles to be enacted in the world. Since then, the government has promoted research and expanded support for individuals with rare and intractable diseases. At first, there were three pillars that were used to clarify causes and treatments: promoting surveys and research; establishing medical institutions; and reducing copayments for medical fees.

In 1995, the Principles of Policy for Rare and Intractable Diseases was revised to include an additional two pillars: improving cooperation between community-based healthcare, medical, and welfare agencies; and promoting welfare measures aimed at improving QOL [4].

The characteristic of *nanbyo* is disease progression, while disability is defined as fixed disorders. Individuals with *nanbyo* had not been recognized as the disabled based on the Act of Services and Supports for Persons with Disabilities. Since this Act was amended in 2013, individuals with *nanbyo* patients have been recognized as the disabled [18]. As a result, the use of disability welfare services (e.g., support consultations, prosthetic devices, and community life support projects) has been expanded to individuals with *nanbyo*.

According to the increasing number of people with intractable diseases, the budget required for medical expense subsidies has also expanded. In addition, from the viewpoint of fairness, there was a demand for the further expansion and review of medical expense subsidies for people with other diseases which had not been defined as the designated *nanbyo*. More than 40 years have elapsed since the establishment of the Principles of Policy for Intractable Disease, and the "law concerning medicine etc. of intractable patients (*nanbyo* law)" [19] has been enforced since January 2015. This *nanbyo* law made stabilized medical expense subsidies by allocating financial resources such as a consumption tax [18, 19]. In addition, the designated *nanbyo* (i.e., the targeted diseases eligible for medical expenses subsidies) has been expanded from 56 diseases to 330 [17].

### 3.3. Social services

Public social services—which *nanbyo* patients can utilize—are gradually increasing. Individuals with *nanbyo* are available to utilize public social services by combining the following four systems: medical insurance, long-term care insurance, the welfare system for persons with disabilities, and the *nanbyo* medical system. Since the different offices deal with each system, it is not easy to use them. However, these four systems are very proud of in the world by the fulfilling contents [19].

Even if healthcare practitioners encourage individuals with *nanbyo* to use social resources, they may be reluctant to initially propose the use of social resources. Multiple factors are implicated in the uptake of social services [20]. 'Internal' issues focused on retaining control and normality within the home. Suggesting an individual use social services can be perceived as insulting because it indicates that the individual cannot provide his or her own medical care good enough or family care is insufficient. Healthcare practitioners must consider the patient's and family's feelings whenever suggesting the use of social services and should research reasonable methods for proposing the use of services.

http://dx.doi.org/10.5772/intechopen.69773

## 4. Home care support system for individuals with ALS

**Figure 3** shows the system for providing home care support during the early stage following diagnosis; **Figure 4** shows the system used during the late and severe stages. The types and frequencies of use for various social services should be considered along with both disease aggravation and the preferences of the individual with ALS and his or her family.

Collaboration among multidisciplinary professionals is extremely important. Because nurses specialize in both medicine and care, they play the role of the glue that holds together the multidisciplinary team [21].

The concept of hope is important to supporting individuals with ALS. Healthcare practitioners need to seek and sustain their hope in individuals with ALS. Individuals with ALS have hope for a cure, social support, searching for information, spiritual beliefs, limiting the impact of the disease, adapting to changing abilities, and self-transcendence [22].

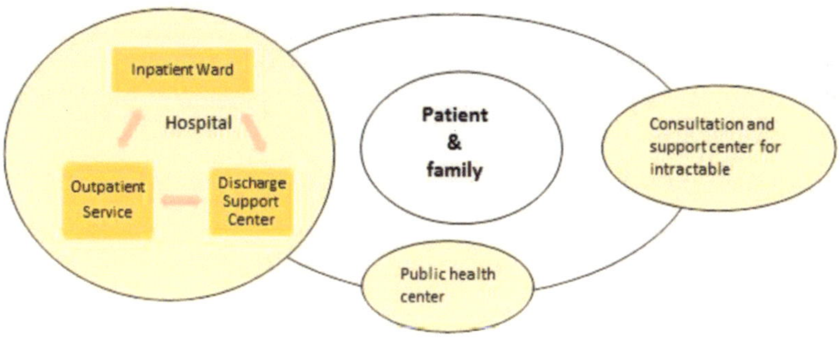


**Figure 3.** Support system for individuals with early stage ALS.

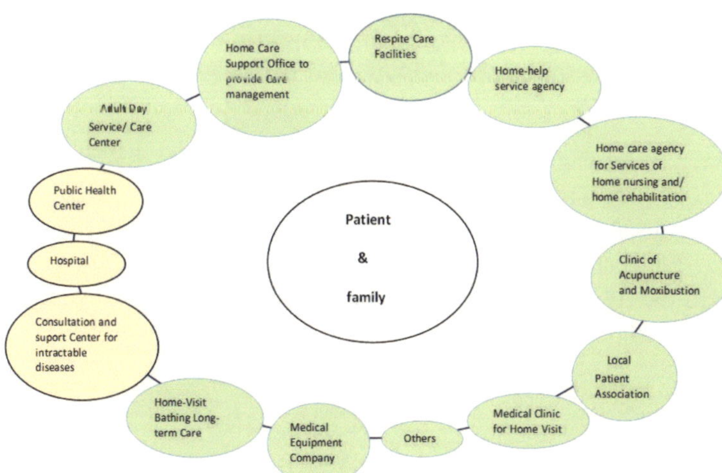


**Figure 4.** Social services and home care support system for the individuals with ALS during disease progression.

## 5. Timely decision-making for medical treatment

Although there is no effective cure for ALS, symptomatic treatment can improve QOL if it is provided in a timely manner. Also, the healthcare provider can modify the illness trajectory, hinder disease progression, and extend survival time. Providing symptomatic treatment is essential in order to gain the patient's understanding and consent. Healthcare practitioners need to understand the reasons why psychological distress of individuals with ALS is generated by social interaction.

Individuals with ALS can hardly accept their diagnosis. As ALS rapidly progresses, their illness acceptance cannot catch up with the reality of disease condition. It is no wonder that patients expect to return their previous health and become well someday, while healthcare practitioners play the percentages based on their knowledge of the disease characteristics. Individuals with ALS suffer from this gap between them and their healthcare practitioners. Also, their families have the poor understanding of the reality of disease progression. This also allows increasing the suffering of the individuals with ALS [23].

Providing information is an important part of decision-making support during disease progression. Healthcare providers consider timing to be a key point in the decision-making process and often postpone decisions until it is not too late.

## 6. End-of-life care in Japan

### 6.1. Two terminal points in individuals with ALS

Individuals with ALS have two terminal points. As respiratory failure worsens, if the patient decides not to receive TPPV, then he or she will die at this primary terminal point. If an individual with ALS selects to receive TPPV at this primary terminal point, he or she will encounter the secondary terminal point at time that TPPV can no longer provide respiratory management.

Ten-year survival rate was 87.1% among individuals with ALS who underwent TPPV from 2000 to 2007 [24]. TPPV allows long-term survival for individuals with ALS, but patients with terminal cancer are limited to live longer even if TPPV is initiated. The other difference between cancer and ALS, as shown in **Figure 5**, is that ALS is living with fear of dying all the time, while cancer patient can change the gear from living positive to death.

### 6.2. Rates of TPPV use

The rate of use of TPPV is higher in Japan than Western countries, as shown in **Table 2**. Some reasons for this discrepancy are summarized in **Table 3**.

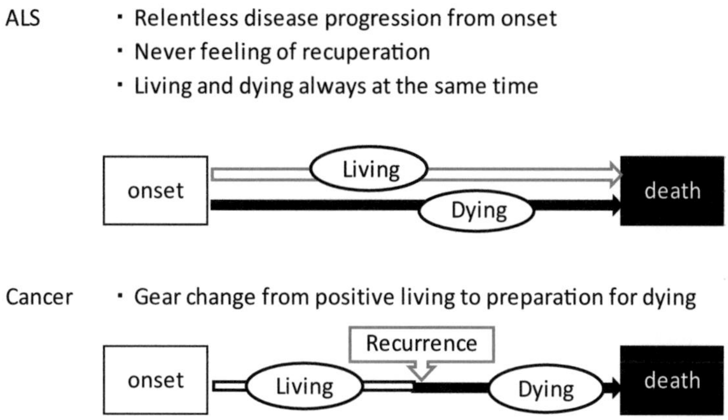


**Figure 5.** Difference between ALS and cancer.

| Citation, which data were requoted | Country | Rate (%) | Study method |
|---|---|---|---|
| Furukawa et al. [25] | Japan | 29.30% | National study |
| | Western countries | 1.5–3.2% | |
| Tagami et al. [26] | Japan and Asian countries | 12.7–21% | |
| | Britain | 0% | A British series of 50 patients |
| | Germany | 3% | |
| | USA | 1.4–14% | |
| | Canada | 1.50% | |
| | France | 2.5–5% | |
| | Norway | 7% for males and 3.8% for females | |
| | Italy | 10.60% | The largest study in north Italy from 1995 to 2004 |
| | Denmark | 22% | |
| Rabkin et al. [27] | USA | 2–6% | |
| | Europe | 0–10.6% | |
| | Japan | 25–46% | |
| Lee et al. [28] | Taiwan | 20.97% | |

**Table 2.** International comparison of TPPV rates.

| Citation | Reasons |
|---|---|
| Tagami et al. [26] | 1. Attributed to religious, ethnic, and cultural differences<br>2. Financial considerations: the Japanese government covers all costs for noninvasive/invasive mechanical ventilation at any age for both inpatients and outpatients<br>3. Regular follow-up examinations at the same institute due to increased availability of continue services and improved knowledge and education regarding ALS<br>4. Peer counseling by the Japanese ALS Association (JALSA)<br>5. Implementation of the long-term care insurance (LTCI) as a new and fundamentally reformed social insurance system at 2000 in Japan |
| Rabkin et al.[27] | Different conceptualizations of the physician's role in medical decision-making, attitudinal differences among patients, caregivers and healthcare professionals and |
| Vianello et al. [29] | 1. To underline a proactive approach by Japanese physicians toward TV<br>2. Traditional fiduciary relationship that exists between the patient and the physician (the traditional Japanese paternalistic medical ethos dictating that "the doctor knows best" associated with physician's belief that patient well-being is the most)<br>3. Be attributable to the contribution offered by family members, given that the family's obligations as home care providers during sickness are deeply embedded in |

**Table 3.** Reasons why Japan has a higher rate of TPPV use than other countries.

### 6.3. High level of disagreement between individuals with ALS and their family members in Japan

Differing opinions about the use of TPPV are often seen between individuals with ALS and their family members. Fifty-four percent of Japanese patients oppose TPPV compared with 10% of Japanese caregivers, but American patients and caregivers show greater agreement in decision-making than their Japanese counterparts [30].

There is no correct answer regarding decision-making. The most important thing on decision-making is what the individual with ALS thinks. However, Japanese individuals with ALS consider the burden of care on their family members to be greater than the burden on themselves and often do not want to receive TPPV. Families want individuals with ALS to receive TPPV because they want their loved ones to live as long as possible. This relationship, which considers each other, results in a large amount of disagreement between the individuals with ALS and their family members.

Having sufficient time to think and discuss will lead to the best decision-making. Healthcare professionals need to promote individuals with ALS discussing decision-making with the relevant family members [31]. Early intervention is necessary before the speech difficulties

http://dx.doi.org/10.5772/intechopen.69773

associated with ALS become severe [30]. A study on American and Canadian patients with ALS reported that advanced directives were in place for 88.9% of patients and followed for 96.8% of patients [32]. However, advanced directives have not been familiarized yet in Japan [33].

| Reference | Published Year | Country | Method | Place of death |
|---|---|---|---|---|
| Gil et al. [35] | 2008 | France | • 302 patients in one of the 16 ALS centers in 15 French regions<br>• Prospective investigation | 63% of patients died in a medical facility |
| Yang et al. [36] | 2011 | China | • 139 patients in West China Hospital of Sichuan Univ.<br>• Survey to family members, caregivers, family physicians | 82% of patients died at home |
| Spataro et al. [37] | 2010 | Italy | • 182 patients in a single ALS tertiary center<br>• Consultation with relatives or family physicians | 85.2% of patients died at home |
| Ushikubo [38] | 2015 | Japan | • 14 patients in users of home care nursing<br>• Interview survey with home care nurses | 43% of patients died at home |
| Dominguez-Berjon et al. [39] | 2015 | Spain | • 1035 in the Autonomous Community of Madrid<br>• A population-based cross-sectional study | 56.1% died in a hospital<br>30.4% at home, 8.3% in a residential home<br>5.1% unknown |
| Escarrabill et al. [41] | 2014 | Portuguese | • 77 from five hospitals<br>• A retrospective medical records analysis | 57% of patients died in a home |
| Tsai et al. [42] | 2013 | Taiwan | • 751 from the National Health Insurance Research Database<br>• A retrospective population-based study | 53.5% died in a medical facility |

**Table 4.** International comparison of the places of death of individuals with ALS.

### 6.4. End-of-life care for patients with ALS receiving NPPV

It is true that palliative end-of-life care for individuals with ALS has not progressed much in Japan [33, 34]. People who use NPPV are increasing because it is a way to palliate respiratory deficiency and give time for decision-making on TPPV. Euthanasia is not legally permitted in Japan. However, NPPV cannot palliate respiratory failure if the disease is severely aggravated [35]. Palliative end-of-life care for patients who choose to remain on NPPV as the ceiling of medical treatment for respiratory failure has received little focus. The development of palliative end-of-life care for ALS patients receiving NPPV is needed [35].

### 6.5. Place of death among individuals with ALS

Understanding the causes and places of death of ALS patients is necessary to develop better end-of-life care. There are seven articles [36–42] that clarify the causes and places of death. The primary cause of death remains respiratory failure. The secondary causes of death vary and include sudden death, death during sleep [38], nutritional causes [37], and cardiovascular diseases [42]. **Table 4** summarizes seven articles on the places of death of individuals with ALS, and these also vary. Age, marital status, and the socioeconomic level of the patient also influence the places of death of patients with ALS [40]. Further research is necessary to develop end-of-life care by elucidating the dying process and analyzing the place of death.

## 7. Conclusion

There is no effective cure for ALS, but symptomatic treatment accomplishes the purpose of palliative care, extends the patient's survival time, and improves their QOL. Healthcare practitioners have many ways to improve illness trajectory and QOL by coping with the various symptoms caused by disease progression in a timely manner. It is important to provide mental care, decision-making support, and family support via multidisciplinary collaboration. Healthcare practitioners make an effort to cherish hope and support the autonomy of the individuals with ALS and their family members. Moreover, it challenges to develop and provide palliative care on the terminal withdrawal of NPPV.

## Author details

Mitsuko Ushikubo

Address all correspondence to: ushi2@gunma-u.ac.jp

Graduate School of Health Sciences, Gunma University, Gunma, Japan

## References

[1] Miller RG, Jackson CE, Kasarskis EJ, England JD, Forshew D, Johnston W, et al. Practice parameter update: The care of the patient with amyotrophic lateral sclerosis: Multidisciplinary care, symptom management, and cognitive/behavioral impairment (an evidence-based review): Report of the Quality Standards, Subcommittee of the American Academy of Neurology. Neurology. 2009;**73**:1227-1233

[2] Bedlack RS, Mitsumoto H, editors. Amyotrophic Lateral Sclerosis: A Patient Care Guide for Clinicians. 1 ed. New York: demosMEDICAL; 2013. pp. 4-14

[3] Ushikubo M, Tomita C, Inokuma A, Ikeda M, Okamoto K. Illness course and circumstances of death among individuals with rapidly progressive amyotrophic lateral sclerosis. International Medical Journal. 2013;**20**(4):446-449

[4] Japan Intractable Disease Information Center. www.nanbyou.or.jp [Internet]. Available from: www.nanbyou.or.jp [Accessed: March 3, 2017]

[5] Doi Y, Atsuta N, Sobue G, Morita M, Nakano I. Prevalence and incidence of amyotrophic lateral sclerosis in Japan. The Journal of Epidemiology. 2014;**24**(6):494-499. DOI: 10.2188/jea.JE20140059

[6] Furuta N, Makioka K, Fujita Y, Okamoto K. Changes in the clinical features of amyotrophic lateral sclerosis in rural Japan. Internal Medicine. 2013;**52**:1691-1696. DOI: 10.2169/internalmedicine.52.0195

[7] Handy CR, Krudy C, Boulis N, Federici T. Pain in amyotrophic lateral sclerosis: A neglected aspect of disease. Neurology Research International. 2011;(403808). DOI: 10.1155/2011/403808

[8] Simmons Z. Management strategies for patients with amyotrophic lateral sclerosis from diagnosis through death. Neurologist. 2005;**11**(5):257-270

[9] Ushikubo M. Shinkei Nanbyo Kanja no Kurushimi ni taisure Kango (nursing to palliate pain and distress of patients with neurological disease). Nanbyo to Zaitaku Kea. 2010;**16**(1):20-23

[10] Ushikubo M. Experiences of individuals living with neuromuscular illness in long course: Palliative care for their psychological distress. Japan Academy of Nursing Science. 2005;**25**(4):70-79

[11] Ogino M. The survey report about the end-of-life care with ALS patients of the ALS physicians in Japan. Clinical Neurology. 2010;**50**:1026-1028

[12] Ministry of Health, Labor and Welfare. Trends in usage of morphine, fentanyl, and oxycodone in Japan; 2011

[13] Yatsumoto K. Palliative care for patients with ALS: Considering the role and involvement of pharmacist. Japanese Journal of Pharmaceutical Palliative Care and Sciences. 2014;**7**:23-28

[14] Grennwood DI. Nutrition management of amyotrophic lateral sclerosis. Nutrition in Clinical Practice. 2013;**28**(3):392-399. DOI: 10.1177/0884533613476554

[15] Chió A, Mora G, Lauria G. Pain in amyotrophic lateral sclerosis. The Lancet Neurology. 2017;**16**:144-156

[16] Saunders CM. The Management of Terminal Malignant Disease. 2nd ed. London: Edward Arnold; 1984. pp. 232-241

[17] Kodama T. Global strategy for rare and intractable diseases. Clinical Neurology. 2013;**53**:1283-1286

[18] Kouno A, editor. Zaitaku Kango Ron (Home Care Nursing). 4th ed. Tokyo: Medical Friend Co.; 2016. pp. 183-194

[19] Kawamura S, Nakayama Y, editors. Nanbyo Kango no Kiso to Jissen (Basic and Practice of Nanbyo Nursing). 1st ed. Tokyo: Kirishobo; 2014. pp. 15-23

[20] O'Brien MR, Whitehead B, Murphy PN, Mitcuhell JD, Jack BA. Social services homecare for people with motor neuron disease/amyotrophic lateral sclerosis: Why are such services used or refused? Palliative Medicine. 2012;**26**(2):121-131. DOI: 10.1177/0269216311398697

[21] Bedlack RS, Mitsumoto H, editors. Amyotrophic Lateral Sclerosis: A Patient Care Guide for Clinicians. New York: demosMedical; 2013. 46 p.

[22] Fanos JH, Gelinas DF, Foster RS, Postone N, Miller RG. Hope in palliative care: from narcissism to self-transcendence in amyotrophic lateral sclerosis. The Journal of Palliative Medicine. 2008;**11**(3):470-475. DOI: 10.1089/jpm.2007.0098.

[23] Ushikubo M. Shinkei nanbyo ryouyousya nitaisuru totaru kea no souzou to hatten (development of total care for people with Nanbyo). Journal of Japan Intractable Illness Nursing. 2009;**14**(2):98-104 (in Japanese)

[24] Nobukuni K, Tanabe Y. Main cause of death and prognosis of ALS patients who underwent TPPV. Nanbyo to Zaitaku Kea. 2010;**16**(1):55-57

[25] Furukawa Y, Komai K, Ishida C, Takahashi K, Takami A, Motozaki Y, et al. Cause of death in Japanese patients with amyotrophic lateral sclerosis on tracheostomy-positive pressure ventilation. European Neurology. 2012;**68**:261-264

[26] Tagami M, Kimura F, Nakajima H, Ishida S, Fujiwara S, Hosokawa T, et al. Tracheostomy and invasive ventilation in Japanese ALS patients: Decision-making and survival analysis: 1990-2010. Journal of the Neurological Sciences. 2014;**344**(158-164)

[27] Rabkin J, Ogino M, Goetz R, Mcihiney M, Hupf J, Heitzuman D, et al. Japanese and American ALS patient preferences regarding TIV: A cross-national survey. Amyotrophic Lateral Sclerosis and Frontotemporal Degeneration. 2014;**15**:185-191

[28] Lee CTC, Ciu Y, Wang KC, Hwang CS, Lin KH, Lin KH, et al. Riluzole and prognostic factors in amyotrophic lateral sclerosis long-term and short-term survival:

A population-based study of 1149 cases in Taiwan. The Journal of Epidemiology. 2013;**23**(1):35-40. DOI: 10.2188/jea.JE20120119

[29] Viaello A, Concas A. Tracheostomy ventilation in ALS: A Japanese bias. The Journal of the Neurological Sciences. 2014;DOI: http://dx.di.org/10.1010/i.jns2014.06.050

[30] Christodoulou G, Goetzu R, Ogino M, Mitsumoto H, Rabkin J. Opinions of Japanese and American ALS caregivers regarding tracheostomy with invasive ventilation (TIV). Amyotrophic Lateral Sclerosis and Frontotemporal Degeneration. 2016;**17**:47-54. DOI:10.3109/21678421.2015.1069850

[31] Ushikubo M, Iida M Ootani T. Nursing support for decision-making of ventilator use in individuals with ALS at home. Kitakanto Medical Journal. 2008;**58**:209-216 (in Japanese)

[32] Mandler RN, Anderson FA Jr, Miller RG, Clawson M, Cudkowicz M, Del Bene M. The ALS patient care database: Insights into end-of-life care in ALS. Amyotrophic Lateral Sclerosis and Other Motor Neuron Disorders. 2001;**2**(4):203-238. DOI: 10.1080/14660820152882214

[33] Hashizumi A, Yamamoto M, Uchiyama T. ALS kanjya san he no jizenishiketteikakun-insyo no unyo to kadai [challenge to implement advance directives to ALS patients]. Nanbyo to Zaitakukea [Nanbyo and home care]. 2007;**13**(4):57-61

[34] Ushikubo M, Okamoto K. Circumstances surrounding death and nursing difficulties with end-of-life care for individuals with ALS in central Japan. International Journal of Palliative Nursing. 2012;**18**(11):554-560

[35] Ushikubo M, Iida M, Suzuki M, Sasaki K. Literature review of palliative end-of-life care for patients with amyotrophic lateral sclerosis under non-invasive positive-pressure ventilation. Kitakanto Medical Journal. 2017;**67**:55-62

[36] Gil J, Funalor B, Verscjierem A, Danel-Brunaud V, Camu W, Vandenberghe N, et al. Causes of death amongst French patients with amyotrophic lateral sclerosis: A prospective study. The European Journal of Neurology. 2008;**15**(11):1245-1251.DOI: 10.1111/j.1468-1331.2008.02307.x

[37] Yang R, Huang R, Chen D, Song W, Zeng Y, Zhao B, et al. Causes and places of death of patients with amyotrophic lateral sclerosis in south-west China. Amyotrophic Lateral Sclerosis. 2011;**12**(3):206-209. DOI: 10.3109/17482968.2011.572979

[38] Spataro R, Lo Re M, Piccoli T, Piccoli F, La Bella V. Causes and place of death in Italian patients with amyotrophic lateral sclerosis. Acta Neurologica Scandinavica. 2010;**122**(3):217-223. DOI: 10.1111/j.1600-0404.2009.01290.x

[39] Ushikubo M. Comparison between home and hospital as the place of death for individuals with amyotrophic lateral sclerosis in the last stages of illness. The American Journal of Hospice and Palliative Medicine. 2015;**32**(4):417-426. DOI: 10.1177/049909114525259

[40] Dominguez-Berjo MF, Esteban-Vasallo MD, Zoni AC, Genova-Maleras R, Astray-Mochales J. Place of death and associated factors among patients with amyotrophic

lateral sclerosis in Madrid (Spain). Amyotrophic Lateral Sclerosis and Frontotemporal Degeneration. 2015;**16**:1-7

[41] Escarrabill J, Vianello A, Farrero E, Ambrosino N, Martinez Llorens J, Vitacca M. Place of death in patients with amyotrophic lateral sclerosis. Revista Portuguesa de Pneumologia. 2014;**20**(4):188-193. DOI: 10.1016/j.rppneu2014.03.001

[42] Tsai CP, Chang BH, Lee CT. Underlying cause and place of death among patients with amyotrophic lateral sclerosis in Taiwan: A population-based study, 2003-2008. The Journal of Epidemiology. 2013;**23**(6):424-428

Chapter 6

# Diabetes, Palliative and End-of-Life Care

Trisha Dunning

Additional information is available at the end of the chapter

http://dx.doi.org/10.5772/67192

**Abstract**

This chapter provides a brief overview of diabetes prevalence, the associated complications, diabetes-related mortality and management strategies to set the context for discussing palliative and end-of-life care. This chapter highlights: (1) The increasing global focus on palliative and end-of life-care; (2) The relationship among health trajectories, function and palliative and end-of-life care; (3) The imperative to plan care with the individual to achieve personalised care that meets the individual's goals, preferences, values and spiritual needs across the various health trajectories; (4) The need to proactively plan for the transition to palliative and end-of-life care when appropriate and while the individual can make informed decisions. Proactively planning for changing care needs is more likely to achieve care consistent with the individual's goals, values and preferences; (5) The key role of family carers and the effect of caring on carers' health; (6) The importance of having timely, meaningful conversations about palliative and end-of-life care with people with diabetes and their families; and (7) The imperative to ameliorate suffering, optimise quality of life and personalising care.

**Keywords:** diabetes, health trajectories, palliative, end-of-life, communication

## 1. Introduction

### 1.1. Diabetes: a significant issue also in palliative care setting

Chronic diseases are the leading cause of death globally [1]. Diabetes is the most prevalent chronic disease affecting 422 million people worldwide [2]. Diabetes is linked to 3.7 million deaths per year [2] and is often associated with other chronic diseases, especially hypertension, cardiovascular disease and renal disease, as well as some forms of cancer. Globally, one person with diabetes dies every six seconds [3].

Most chronic disease-related deaths occur in older age and are associated with potentially remediable physical, emotional and spiritual suffering [4].Relief from suffering is more likely to be achieved if palliative care is initiated early [5]. In addition, early initiation of palliative care leads to cost savings [4]. Significantly, outcomes for people who receive early palliative care are better than those who receive 'usual' care [6]. Consequently, the management of diabetes and its complications is a significant issue to be addressed early in the course of the disease and also in palliative care settings.

People with diabetes are living longer; but diabetes is associated with 8–11% lower 5–10 years survival rates [7]. However, older people with diabetes are a heterogeneous population and there are different types of risks within the population. Several interrelated factors affect survival: duration of diabetes >12 years, poor glycaemic control, multiple comorbidities (comorbid load), especially cardiovascular disease and heart failure, end stage renal failure, advanced foot disease and frailty.

Polypharmacy confers an increased mortality risk for people with diabetes through the interactions among medicines and individual medicine side effects. For example, thiazolidinedione glucose lowering medicines are linked to heart failure and other cardiovascular mortality [8]. Insulin and sulphonylureas are linked to adverse outcomes in older people with diabetes and mortality [9, 10]. Currie et al. [9] described mortality hazard between 10 and 34% for these medicines in combination with metformin and even higher levels when they were used as monotherapy. Glycaemic control is important with good control, HbA1c, <7% (53 mmol/mol) conferring benefits. However, hypoglycaemia is associated with risk of cardiac changes and death, especially in older people and can occur when HbA1c is high as well as low [11].

These risks highlight the importance of identifying and managing the factors that affect mortality as early as possible in the health trajectory, see Section 6. Individually and collectively, they are associated with increased costs, unnecessary interventions, including in the late stages of life, and consequent physical and mental suffering for people with diabetes and families. They also need to be considered and managed in palliative care settings.

## 2. Managing diabetes

Diabetes management requires interdisciplinary team care. Collaborative, respectful interdisciplinary care predicated on effective communication is essential when palliative and end-of-life care is indicated. Diabetes education is regarded as the cornerstone of management and is essential to enable the individual to undertake self-care such as blood glucose monitoring, managing medicines and attending health professional appointments to achieve good outcomes. Education about palliative care options and planning for end-of-life care are not currently regarded as core aspects of diabetes education. However, these issues should be discussed as the person's health and functional status (trajectory) changes.

Eating a healthy diet, regular physical activity/exercise and managing stress (lifestyle factors) are key management strategies for all types of diabetes and for people of all ages, including when glucose lowering medicines (GLM) and other medicines are required [12]. Healthy active lifestyle also helps protect telomeres and overall health [13].

The broad aim of diabetes management is to keep the blood glucose and HbA1c (an indicator of the average blood glucose level over 3 months) as close to the normal range as possible to prevent or manage long-term diabetes complications. Such complications are associated with reduced life expectancy. However, the blood glucose and HbA1c range must be safe for the individual depending on their functional category, disease trajectory and life expectancy [12, 15].

The risk of severe hypoglycaemia increases, if HbA1c and blood glucose ranges are near or lower than normal in people with multiple comorbidities, longer duration of diabetes and those on insulin/sulphonylureas [11]. Hypoglycaemia is associated with other risks such as falls. Hyperglycaemia can also contribute to falls cognitive changes and delirium. Example HbA1c and blood glucose ranges are as follows:

### 2.1. HbA1c

- In healthy people with short duration of diabetes, no cardiovascular disease, and no severe hypoglycaemia, the HbA1c range is 6.5–7.0% (48–53 mmol/mol). The focus is on preventing complications [3, 14, 15].
- In frail older people with complication's and comorbidities, limited life expectancy and those at the end-of-life, the HbA1c range is 8–8.5% (64–69 mmol/mol). The focus is on managing existing complications to promote safety (palliative approach) [3, 14, 15].

### 2.2. Blood glucose

- Healthy people with type 2 diabetes (T2DM): fasting 6–8, postprandial 6–10 mmol/L [15].
- Frail older people, those with dementia and those with high hypoglycaemia risk on GLMs 6–11 mmol/L [15].

Thus, the management focus and the metabolic parameters used to determine the effective ness of management strategies often need to change as function and the health trajectory change [16, 17]. Palliative care is a valuable care option, however, many people who would benefit from palliative care to manage symptoms and reduce suffering are not offered such care because health professionals underestimate the problem and are often reluctant to discuss the issue or to give 'bad news' [17]. People with life limiting illnesses should not be excluded from potentially beneficial treatment.

Palliative care can be used for seriously ill surgical patients, and preoperative screening for frailty can reduce 180 days mortality [18]. Likewise, a systematic review of 25 paper involving 8575 patients and 22 different interventions suggests preoperative decision-making concerning palliative care can improve communication, symptom management and reduce use of health care resources and costs [19]. More research is required to substantiate these findings due to methodological flaws and differences and small sample sizes in many of the papers included in the review.

## 3. Glucose lowering medicines

The main types of GLMs are shown in **Table 1**.

Medicines, including GLMs, play a key role in diabetes management in all health trajectories. Medicines confer significant benefits, but they are also associated with adverse events, including in palliative care settings. Ageing and diabetes-related pathophysiological changes and their subsequent risks significantly affect medicine safety and medicine choices and increase the risk of medicine-related adverse events [20]. As people with diabetes grow older, or develop dementia, they have difficulty managing their medicines and rely on other people to help them manage their medicines and other diabetes self-care and activities of daily living. Difficulty managing medicines is one reason for admission to a care home [20].

Key changes that affect medicine action, effectiveness and safety include:

- cardiovascular changes, which affect medicines distribution
- liver changes, which affects medicine metabolism
- renal disease, which affects excretion
- gastrointestinal changes that affect absorption of oral medicines
- changes in the counter-regulatory response to hypoglycaemia due to reduced production of glucagon and autonomic neuropathy, which cause hypoglycaemic unawareness
- cognitive and sensory changes, which affects independence and medicine adherence.

Polypharmacy is common in people with diabetes, especially people with type 2 diabetes who have comorbidities. Polypharmacy might be indicated to manage symptoms and comorbidities, but it is important to use non-medicine options where possible and to ensure polypharmacy is 'thoughtful'. That is, where possible medicines should be stopped before starting another medicine and not commencing medicines whose benefits take longer than the person's life expectancy [20]. The risks and benefits of each medicine must be considered individually, and in the context of the whole medicine regimen, and the individual's goals, preferences and values [21, 22].

Diabetogenic medicines such as corticosteroids, antipsychotics and thiazide diuretics can contribute to hyperglycaemia and induce diabetes in previously undiagnosed older people [3, 15]. High dose corticosteroids are often used in cancer to manage symptoms, cachexia and poor appetite.

### 3.1. Hypoglycaemia

Changes in pancreatic alpha cells with increasing duration of diabetes and advancing age affects glucagon production, which reduces the individual's ability to mount an effective counter-regulatory response to hypoglycaemia [22–24]. In addition, autonomic and sensory changes affect the individual's ability to recognise the usual hypoglycaemic autonomic

http://dx.doi.org/10.5772/67192

| Type of medicine | Main mode of action | Main side effects |
|---|---|---|
| **Oral GLMs** | | |
| Metformin | Reduces hepatic glucose output. | Gastrointestinal (GIT) problems such as bloating and flatulence in the early days.<br>GIT problems less likely with slow release dose forms (these should not be crushed).<br>Rarely lactic acidosis—contraindicated in significant renal failure.<br>Long-term use might lead to vitamin $B_{12}$ deficiency and lead to anaemia and its consequences. |
| Sulphonylureas | Binds to the beta cell receptor and triggers insulin release independent of glucose. | Hypoglycaemia.<br>Weight gain. |
| DPP-4 inhibitors | Improve beta cell function and insulin secretion. Reduces gastric emptying and postprandial blood glucose. | GIT problems.<br>Nasopharyngitis.<br>Heart failure in people with or at risk of cardiovascular disease. |
| Thiazolidinediones (TZD) | Sensitise tissues to insulin. | Weight gain.<br>Fluid retention.<br>Heart failure.<br>Risk of non-axial fracture in women |
| Alpha-glucosidase inhibitor | Slows carbohydrate absorption from the intestines and reduces postprandial blood glucose. | GIT problems especially bloating and flatulence. |
| Sodium-glucose cotransporter-2 (SGLT-2) | Inhibit the SGLT-2 transporter exchange sodium and glucose in the kidney and glucose is excreted in the urine.<br>Reduces systolic blood pressure and cardiovascular risk. | Dehydration.<br>Dizziness.<br>Risk of genitourinary infections.<br>Older people risk of electrolyte changes and hyperosmolar states.<br>Not use with loop diuretics. |
| **Injectable GLMs** | | |
| GLP-1 | | Weight loss<br>GIT problems especially nausea and vomiting |
| Insulin*<br>Short, rapid, intermediate and long acting analogues<br>Premixed | Lower blood glucose | Hypoglycaemia |

**Notes:** *Injecting repeatedly into the same site can cause lipodystrophy and lipoatrophy. Injecting in lipodystrophy/atrophy tissue or using incorrect injection technique or needle size can affect insulin action and effectiveness and lead to glucose variability [51].

Combinations of some types of oral GLMs and of the different types of insulin are available.

**Table 1.** Classes of glucose lowering medicines, main mode of action and main side effects.

warning symptoms (sweating, trembling and palpitations) and put them at significant risk of severe hypoglycaemia requiring hospital admission, and cardiovascular complications [25].

A severe hypoglycaemia is associated with poor prognosis, leads to cognitive changes, coma, falls and injuries such as fractures, cognitive changes, acute coronary syndrome, recurrent hypoglycaemia, admission to hospital and sudden death [22, 23]. Hypoglycaemia affects age-related cognitive function due to changes in the counter-regulatory response to hypoglycaemia and the delivery of 'fuel' to the brain. Executive function is affected and reduces the individual's ability to recognise, problem-solve, make decisions, including about treating their hypoglycaemia [26] and is associated with dementia in the long term [27]. In addition, hypoglycaemia engenders fear, reduces quality of life (QOL) of the individual and family caregivers [28].

### 3.2. Hyperglycaemia

Hyperglycaemia is not a benign condition. It is an underlying cause of complications that affect functional status and life expectancy [3, 15]. It causes unpleasant symptoms and other metabolic changes such as incontinence, dehydration, triggers inflammatory processes, increases risk of intercurrent infections, weight loss and affects cognitive function. Some of these processes can lead to ketoacidosis (DKA) in type 1 diabetes (T1DM) and hyperglycaemia hyperosmolar states (HHS) in T2DM [3, 14, 15].

## 4. Palliative care

Palliative care was traditionally used to refer to care of people at the end-of-life. Definitions of palliative, end-of-life and terminal care are shown in **Table 2**. It is important to note that the definition of palliative care changed over 6 years ago to encompass chronic diseases that have a longer trajectory to end-of-life [29]. The definition was changed to reflect the association among chronic disease, suffering and life expectancy, and the fact that the chronic disease and frailty trajectories to death are less predictable than and different from the cancer trajectory. Health trajectories are described in Section 6.

As indicated, palliative care improves function and QOL and reduces unwanted hospital admissions and aggressive end-of-life care. It can be delivered in various settings such as in individual's homes, hospital, aged care homes and hospices. Palliative care can be integrated with usual diabetes care including at diagnosis, or can replace usual care.

Palliative care is associated with improved outcomes if it is implemented early; but most people are not referred to palliative care services until last few weeks of life [29, 30] and are often admitted to and die in intensive care units, despite meeting Gold Standards Framework (GSF) criteria [31]. Significantly, older people often meet medical emergency team (MET) criteria before they are discharged from hospital and often represent 30 days of discharge or sooner [32].

MET criteria refer to vital signs such as blood pressure, respiration and heart rate and rhythm that are monitored to detect change to enable treatment to be implemented to prevent a medical

| | |
|---|---|
| **Palliative care** | Palliative care is predicated on the fact that dying is a normal process. It focuses on improving quality of life by relieving suffering, promoting comfort and managing symptoms through comprehensive assessments and personalising care by engaging with the individual and family carers. Palliative care can be integrated with usual diabetes care at any stage in the disease trajectory. Most benefits accrue when palliative care is introduced early. It emphasises the importance of counselling patients and families, supporting patients to understand the change in the focus of care and helping them make decisions about their treatment and goals of care, documenting their end-of-life care preferences and care coordination. |
| **Advance care planning** | The process patients, family members or surrogate decision-makers and health professionals anticipate, discuss, document and communicate treatment options as the health status changes. Advance care plans help health professionals make 'in the moment decisions', which can be emotionally confronting, especially when there is conflict within the family. |
| **End-of-life care** | End-of-life care refers care for likely to die in the following 12 months. It includes imminent death in a few hours or days and progressive incurable life-threatening illnesses such as diabetes. |
| **Terminal care** | Last few days or hours of life. |

**Table 2.** Definitions of palliative care, advance care planning and end-of-life care and terminal care [29, 35, 36].

emergency. Worryingly, 25% of people are discharged *on the same day they have a MET call* [33], and 30% of people aged 70 and 50% of those aged 80 and older leave hospital more disabled then when they were admitted. Recognising and responding to deterioration is essential [34] to treat remedial deterioration as soon as possible. Blood glucose monitoring can be a useful tool to detect deterioration associated with hypo- and hyperglycaemia and implement treatment before preventable conditions such as DKA and HHS. That is, the health trajectory and life expectancy can change during and after a hospital admission.

### 4.1. Goals of palliative care

The main goals of palliative care are to:

- Improve and maintain function to support independence and QOL.
- Achieve their life goals.
- Remain comfortable and free of pain and distressing symptoms.
- Achieve a dignified death in their place of choice.
- Address their spiritual, cultural and religious needs.

These goals also apply to individuals with diabetes [3, 35, 36]. They highlight the importance of discussing life and care goals, values and preferences with people with diabetes and ensuring they are documented and communicated to the family and the individual's other clinicians. Clinicians need to accept that the individual may have different views from their own, and often from their family. In addition, people can change their care preferences over time; therefore, clinicians should ask about any changes for time-to-time such as during annual health reviews, preoperative assessments and changes in health status.

It is also important to provide support for families and other caregivers, including after the death of a loved one when they are particularly vulnerable to acute cardiovascular events, infection and depression [3, 38, 39].

### 4.2. Health trajectories

The complex changing nature of diabetes and prognostic uncertainty makes it difficult to predict when an individual with diabetes would benefit from palliative care. Understanding their functional status and health trajectory can enable health professionals to discuss future care including the option of palliative care and to commence planning for the end-of-life. The following health trajectories are a useful framework for monitoring current and changing health status and care needs and to plan care with people with diabetes to meet changing needs [40, 41].

Unintentional injuries in older people, especially falls, often lead to death and can occur in any health trajectory.

1. **Trajectory 1**: Health trajectory where the person is independent, and has none or few complications when the focus is on maintaining health and preventing complications by striving for normoglycaemia (tight glycaemic control). However, death can be sudden in diabetes due to hypoglycaemia or silent myocardial infarction.

2. **Trajectory 2**: Sometimes called the cancer trajectory. There is a steady reasonably predictable decline in physical health over time (weeks, months or years). However, some cancers are curable and people may survive for many years and are referred to as cancer survivors. That is, they enter another health trajectory.

3. **Trajectory 3**: It is associated with long-term functional decline and intermittent periods of deterioration (unstable diabetes, e.g., due to intercurrent illness) that can be serious and require admission to hospital and/or intensive care unit (ICU). The individual usually recovers, but each deterioration results in further decline and can result in death. The time of death is unpredictable. Older people admitted to ICU are likely to die and may derive more benefit from palliative care, which avoids unnecessary life-prolonging treatment. Generally, QOL and pain management are more important to people with limited life expectancy than prolonging life.

4. **Trajectory 4**: People who do not have cancer or chronic diseases that cause organ damage/failure are likely to die at an older age from dementia or generalised frailty that involves multiple body systems after 'prolonged dwindling'.

Physical, psychological and spiritual needs differ among people with diabetes and their families and among and within the trajectories. Therefore, palliative and end-of-life care plans should be developed sensitively and reviewed regularly to ensure they reflect the preferences of the individual [35, 40, 42]. Cultural and religious beliefs and traditions about health/ill health, death and dying must be considered and respected, including care of the body after death. **Table 3** shows some assessment and screening tools that can be used to monitor the individual's trajectory.

Malnutrition, deficient calorie, vitamin, mineral, protein, water intake, contributes to frailty and 'failure to thrive' in older people described in trajectory 4 [43]. Failure to thrive is associated with weight loss, often dehydration, skin fragility, osteoporosis, depression, immune system dysfunction, low cholesterol and functional decline [43]. Diabetes complications affect the individual's ability to thrive, as do some medicines. It is present in 5–35% of community dwelling older Americans, 25–40% of older people in aged care homes and increases the risk of morbidity and mortality. Palliative can be very valuable in such people.

It is generally difficult to precisely predict when an individual will die. Prognosis prediction models and their clinical utility in palliative care are addressed in a dedicated chapter of this book.

Some general indicators of poor prognosis are described in the Gold Standards Framework (GSF) [31] and can also inform care decisions, for example:

- Sarcopenia and frailty.
- Hospital admissions—increased risk of death in people >65 years with mulitmorbidities and heart failure.
- Sentinel events such as a fall, bereavement, and admission to and aged care home.
- Serum albumin <2.5 g/dL.
- Weight loss >10% in the preceding 6 months, although some experts indicate weight loss >5% over 6 months should be investigated.

Another useful prognostic indicator is the 'surprise question': would I be surprised if this person died in the next 12 months? If the answer is 'no, I would not be surprised', it is time to discuss and document palliative and end-of-life care, if that has not already been done [31, 41]. Documented palliative/end-of-life care plans should be reviewed. If the answer is 'yes' it could be time to begin initiating health professional and family case conferences.

Physical, psychological and spiritual needs differ among people with diabetes and their families and among and within the trajectories. As indicated, palliative and end-of-life care plans should be reviewed regularly to ensure they reflect the preferences of the individual. Cultural and religious beliefs and traditions about health/ill health, death and dying must be considered and respected including care of the body after death. The risk of developing many diseases increase with age, including diabetes, dementia and some forms of cancer; 80% of cancers occur after age 60 [44]. Some cancers and type 2 diabetes are associated with obesity [45]. Thus, it is reasonable to expect the health trajectory to change over time.

| Tool | Comments |
|---|---|
| The surprise question *Would I be surprised if this person died within 12 months?* | Ask any time health changes. |
| Gold Standard Framework (GSF) prognostic indicator guidance | General indicators of decline/deterioration and the increasing need or choice for no further active care. Includes the surprise question. |
| Cognitive assessment toolkit<br>Mini-mental examination | Assess cognitive function. |
| Supportive and palliative care indicators tool (SPICT) | Identify people at risk of deteriorating and dying. |
| Palliative care necessities CCOMS-ICO (NECPAL) | Identify people in need of palliative care. |
| RADboud indicators for palliative care needs (RADPAC) | Identify indicators of palliative care needs. |
| Charlson comorbidity index (CCI) | Designed to estimate 1–10 years mortality in longitudinal studies but is not a valid prognostic indicator for short term outcomes. |
| Clinical frailty scale | Determine frailty and function. |
| Karnofsky performance status scale | Quality of life across the spectrum of health from well to terminal. |
| Barthel index | Assesses capacity to perform basic activities of daily living. |
| Confusion assessment method (CAM) | Determine presence of confusion. |
| Weight, body mass index, food records, and nutrition assessment tools | Monitor nutrition status and related risk of malnutrition. |
| Hypoglycaemia risk assessment tool | Determine risk of hypoglycaemia. Available in the McKellar Guidelines www.adma.org.au/…/133-the-mckellar-guidelines-for-managing-older-people-with-diabetes-in-residential-and-other-care-settings_9dec2013 |
| Diabetes-specific medicine-related adverse risk assessment tool | Determine risk of medicine-related adverse events. Available in the McKellar Guidelines |
| Medicine-related tools, e.g., Beers and STOPP/START | Used when prescribing medicines, when new symptoms develop and to undertake regular medicine reviews. When any new medicines is commenced and new symptoms develop especially in older people. |
| Absolute cardiovascular risk benefit calculator | Estimate cardiovascular risk including when prescribing medicines. |
| Fracture risk assessment tool (FRAX) | Estimate risk of fracture including when frail and when prescribing medicines. |
| Acute physiology and chronic disease evaluation (APACHE) and its variants | Designed to measure severity of disease in adults and used to predict in-hospital death and risk-adjusted length of stay in ICU.<br>Indicate risk of death in patient groups rather than specific individuals and depend on laboratory data. |

**Table 3.** Some useful assessment/screening tools can be used in any health trajectory.

http://dx.doi.org/10.5772/67192

## 5. Personalised palliative, end-of-life care and advance care planning

It is essential to actively involve people in decisions about their care goals, targets and plan including commencing and stopping medicines and other treatments. Involving people in care decisions can be challenging for many health professionals, especially when it concerns emotive issues such as palliative and end-of-life care. Well-designed training courses can improve health professional communication skills [32]. Health professionals find it difficult to resolve the dilemma among 'truth telling', instilling hope, and respecting people's autonomy. Truth telling often means delivering 'bad news' and is stressful. Thus, despite the global trend towards 'truth telling', non-disclosure is still an issue [29, 45].

People with a life-threatening illness (and their families) often ask 'how long have I got?' Inherent in that question is recognition that they have a life-threatening illness and need some guidance about the likely health trajectory (what will happen?), so they can complete 'unfinished business and get their house in order'. They may not initiate discussion about the issue, often because they do not want to upset family, friends or their health professionals. In most cases, people are not concerned so much about dying, as they are of suffering, and having loved ones witness their suffering [38, 46].

Most people want to die at home and die with dignity [29, 30]. Several resources and decision aids are available to help people with diabetes and health professionals make care decision by helping them decide an individual's personal risks and leads to the appropriate use of elective procedures [47]. Some useful resources are listed after the reference list.

### 5.1. Advance care planning

Various countries have different legislative and other procedures guiding advance care planning. Such planning involves shared responsibility among health professionals, the individual and their families. The aim is to identify the individual's values, preferences and goals and communicate them to relevant services and relevant others so the plan can be implemented when indicated.

Research shows people with cancer and dementia have a better end-of-life quality than those with end stage renal disease, cardiopulmonary failure and frailty [29, 30]. Some possible reasons include early initiation of palliative care, documented advance care plans, 'not for resuscitation orders', and fewer admissions to ICU [32, 47]. These findings suggest it is imperative that other disease processes ensure palliative and end-of-life care planning are included in clinical management guidelines.

Key information to discuss and document includes preferences concerning:

- Resuscitation
- Airway support
- Enteral nutrition and fluids

- MET calls if they are admitted to hospital
- Pain management
- Diabetes self-care such as blood glucose monitoring and GLMs
- Other important end-of-life planning includes religious, spiritual and cultural issues surrounding end-of-life care, making a will, funeral planning and designating surrogate decision-makers/power of attorney.

## 6. Good communication

Communication is central to effective palliative care planning. Listening, effective use of silence and using appropriate probing and clarifying questions are key clinician skills [46]. A variety of communication strategies have been designed to enhance health professional and people with diabetes capacity to discuss these emotive issues in a timely and sensitive manner and help reduce uncertainty. However, decisions about treatment options are increasingly complex in an age where advanced technology and treatments promise the hope of extending life.

Initiating discussion about end-of-life care earlier and in a planned manner enables people to make more informed choices when they are not under physical or mental stress and achieve better outcomes. People who discuss their palliative and end-of-life care needs are more likely to receive care consistent with those preferences [6, 29, 30]. Such discussion includes clarifying the individual's goals and their concept of what a 'good death' means to them. Health professionals need to have the relevant skills to communicate about these issues.

## 7. Family carers

Family carers, often a spouse, play a significant role supporting and caring for people with diabetes. They often have health problems themselves and are at high risk of unexpected morbidity and mortality after the death of a loved one, especially if the death is unexpected and not planned for [37, 38]. Caring is hard work and often causes stress that affects sleep, immunity and wellbeing and mobilises inflammatory processes and haemodynamic changes that predispose them to dying [37]. The family carer can neglect their own health care such as taking medicines to perform the caring role. Therefore, carers also need a care plan and their health needs to be monitored. Keeping carers informed and included in case conferences and care decision can reduce stress.

A significant cause of family stress the uncertainties associated with dying. These include undertaking diabetes management tasks such as blood glucose monitoring and injecting insulin and understanding when their loved one is actively dying [46]. Family are often reluctant to support loved ones die at home because of these uncertainties and the responsibility involved. Ensuring these issues are included in family discussions can help relieve stress. Significantly, carer wellbeing affects the experiences of the person they provide care for. The latter are likely to report poor quality of life if their carer has depression [47]. Thus, carers can be 'invisible' or 'hidden' patients.

http://dx.doi.org/10.5772/67192

## 8. What do people with diabetes think?

People with diabetes and their health professionals face many complex decisions where there is no right or wrong answer when considering palliative and end-of-life care. Prognostic uncertainty, competing priorities and weighing benefits and risks overall and the positive and negative outcomes of treatment complicate decision-making [30]. Such decisions can be particularly challenging with respect to managing diabetes when the focus on tight blood glucose control no longer confers benefit and changes to focusing on safety comfort and quality of life, especially given there are no large observational or randomised controlled trials to support many care recommendations [40].

We interviewed people with diabetes receiving palliative care for a range of diagnoses, their family carers (mostly spouses) and palliative care health professionals when we developed Guidelines for Managing Diabetes at the End of Life [35]. Our research suggests people with diabetes and families regard blood glucose testing as an important guide to detecting hypo- and hyperglycaemia, both of which compromise comfort [47, 48]. It is also a reassuringly familiar routine in a sometimes rapidly changing world.

People with diabetes indicated health professionals do not pay enough attention to their diabetes, do not understand the physical and psychological impact of hypo- and hyperglycaemia and the relentless self-care required to manage diabetes and do not respect their lifetime of accumulating diabetes knowledge and solving diabetes care problems. Generally, they wanted blood glucose monitoring continued until the final stages of dying because 'it helps sort out the causes of things like confusion and pain' [47]. They also wanted to continue taking their GLMs until the terminal stage to manage hyperglycaemia, which they stated caused confusion, frequency and tiredness, what affected their comfort and quality of life.

Carers were interviewed separately and reported similar views. They also reported they worried about having to undertake diabetes tasks such as blood glucose testing and administering insulin because they had not received education about these tasks and worried that they might accidently give the wrong insulin dose and hasten death [47, 48].

Our earlier research indicated health professionals reported dilemmas deciding when 'is the right time, to stop blood glucose monitoring and felt finger pricking caused discomfort. They felt 'there was a tension between avoiding discomfort and performing useful investigations' [49]. This study was the impetus for developing the Guidelines for Managing Diabetes at the End of Life [35], which as currently under review.

## 9. Summary

Proactively planning for palliative and end-of-life care can improve comfort and other outcomes for people with diabetes, especially in older age, and their families. Planning for the end-of-life is a shared responsibility between health professionals, people with diabetes and often family carers and reduces decisional conflict when health deteriorates. It is essential to understand people's goals, values and preferences and to personalise care. It is important to consider culture and religion and proactively monitor the individual's and their families' health status. Palliative care aims to promote comfort and alleviate suffering (see **Table 2**) It can be initiated at any time in the diabetes trajectory: early initiation results in better outcomes. General palliative and end-of-life care/guidelines discussed in other chapters in the book apply to people with diabetes. This chapter addressed key diabetes-related care issues that need to be considered.

Significantly: *The way people dies remains in the memory of those who live on.* [Dame Cecily Saunders] [50].

## Author details

Trisha Dunning

Address all correspondence to: trisha.dunning@barwonhealth.org.au

Centre for Quality and Patient Safety Research, School of Nursing and Midwifery, Deakin University and Barwon Health Partnership, Geelong, Victoria, Australia

## References

[1] Centre for Disease Control and Prevention. Chronic Disease Prevention and Health Promotion [Internet]. 2016. Available from: www.cdc.gov/CD/ [Accessed: November 2016]

[2] World Health Day [Internet]. 2016. Available from: www.ibtimes.co.uk/world-health-day-2016-facts-figures-statistics-about-diabetes-1553515

[3] International Diabetes' Federation (IDF). Global Guideline for Managing Older People with Type 2 Diabetes [Internet]. 2013. Available from: www.idf.org [Accessed: January 2016]

[4] Lyness J. End-of-life care: Issues related to geriatric psychiatry. FOCUS Journal Lifelong Learning in Psychiatry. 2005;**3**(2):334-353

[5] Advisory Bard Company. Realising the Full Benefit of Palliative Care [Internet]. 2013. Available from: www.advisory.com [Accessed: January 2016]

[6] Temel J. When more is not better: How to integrate goals of care in conversations about stopping chemotherapy. In: Proceedings of the American Society of Clinical Oncology Annual Meeting; Chicago, Illinois, Journal of Clinical Oncology. May 29 2015

[7] Barnett K, Mcmurdo M, Ogston S, Morris A, Evans J. Mortality in people diagnosed with type 2 diabetes at an older age: a systematic review. Age and Ageing. 2006;**35**:463-468

[8] Singh S, Loke, Y, Furberg C. Thiazolidinediones and heart failure: A teleo-analysis. Diabetes Care. 2017;**30**:2148-2153

[9] Currie C, Poole C, Evans M, Peters J, Morgan C. Mortality and other important diabetes-related outcomes with insulin vs other antihyperglycemic therapies in type 2 diabetes. Journal Clinical Endocrinology Metabolism. 2013;**98**(2):668-677. DOI: 10.1210/jc.2012-304

[10] Mogensen U, Andersson C, Fosbøl E, Schramm T, Vaag A, Scheller N, Torp-Pedersen C, Gislason G, Køber L. Metformin in combination with various insulin secretagogues in type 2 diabetes and associated risk of cardiovascular morbidity and mortality--a retrospective nationwide study. Diabetes Research Clinical Practice 2015;**107**(1):104-112. DOI: 10.1016/j.diabres.2014.09.047

[11] Grembowski D, Ralston J, Anderson M. Hemoglobin A1c, comorbid conditions and all-cause mortality in older patients with diabetes mellitus: A retrospective 9-year cohort study. Diabetes Research Clinical Practice 2014;**106**(2):373-382

[12] American Diabetes Association. Standards of Care [Internet]. 2016. Available from: www.diabetes.org/.../clinical-practice-recommendations%20

[13] Shammas M. Telomeres, lifestyle, cancer and aging. Current Opinion in Clinical Nutrition Metabolic Care. 2011;**14**(1):26-34

[14] Dhaliwal R, Weinstock R. Management of type 1 diabetes in older adults. Diabetes Spectrum. 2014;**27**(1):9-20

[15] Dunning T, Savage S, Duggan N. The McKellar Guidelines for Managing Older People with Diabetes in Residential and Other Care Settings [Internet]. 2013. Available from: www.adma.org.au/.../133-the-mckellar-guidelines-for-managing-older-people-with-diabetes-in-residential-and-other-care-settings_9dec2013 [Accessed: January 2016]

[16] Zheng L, Finucane A, Oxenham D. How good is primary care at identifying patients who need palliative care? A mixed methods study. European Journal Palliative Care. 2013;**20**(5):216-222

[17] Claessen S, Francke A, Engles Y, Deliens L. How do GPs identify a need for palliative care in their patients? An interview study BMC Family Practice. 2013;**14**:42

[18] Ernst K, Hall D, Schmid K. Surgical palliative care consultations over time in relationship to systemwide fraily screening. JAMA Surgery. 2014;**149**(11):1121-1126

[19] Lilley E, Khan K, Johnston F. Palliative care interventions for surgical patients: A systematic review. Journal of the American Medical Association Surgery. 2016;**15**(2):172-183

[20] Matlow J, Bronskill S, Gruneir A, Bell C, Stall N, Herrmann N,Seitz D, Gill S, Austin P, Fischer H, Fung K, Wu W, Rochon P. Use of medications of questionable benefit at end of life in nursing home residents with advanced dementia. JACS Clinical Investigation. March 29 2017. DOI: 10.111/jgs.14844

[21] Institute of Medicine (US) Committee on Care at the End of Life' Approaching death; Improving Care at the End of Life. Washingtong DC: National Academic Press; 1997

[22] Dorman Marek K, Antle L. Chapter 18, Medication management of the community-dwelling older adult. Patient safety and quality: An Evidence-based Handbook for Nurses. 2008;1-38

[23] Seaquist E, Anderson J, Childs B, Cryer P. What are the limitations of hypoglycaemia on both short and long term outcomes in people with diabetes? Diabetes Care. 2013;**35**(5):1384-1395

[24] Meneilly G, Cheung E, Tuokko H. Counter-regulatory hormone responses to hypoglycaemia in elderly patients with diabetes. Diabetes. 2011;**43**(3):403-410

[25] Chopra S, Kewal A. Does hypoglycaemia cause cardiovascular events? Indian Journal Endocrinology and Metabolism. 2012;**16**(1):102-104

[26] McNaf E. The impact of recurrent hypoglycaemia on cognitive function in ageing. Neurobiology Ageing. 2005;**26**(Supp 1):76-79

[27] Yaffe C, Fulvey C, Hamilton M. Association between hypoglycaemia and dementia in a biracial cohort of older adults with diabetes mellitus. JAMA Internal Medicine. 2013;**173**(14):1300-1306

[28] Cox D, Goner-Frederick L, Nowacek G, Butterfield J. Fear of hypoglycaemia: Quantifying, validation and utilization, Diabetes Care. 1987;**10**(5):617-612

[29] Worldwide Palliative Care Alliance (WPCA)/World Health Organisation (WHO). 2014. Available from: www.THEWPCA.org

[30] Sweriessen H, Duckett S. Dying Well: The Grattan Report. 2014. ISBN:1-925015-81-4

[31] Gold Standards Framework Centre. Prognostic Indicator Guidance [Internet]. 2011. Available from: http://www.goldstandardsframework.org.uk/cd-contemt/uploads/files/General%Files/Prognostic%20Indicator%20Guidance%20October%201011.pdf [Accessed: December 2016]

[32] Milnes S, Orford N, Berkeley L, Lambert N, Simpson N, Elderkin T, Corke C, Bailey M. A prospective observational study of prevalence and outcomes of patients with Gold Standard Framework criteria in a tertiary regional Australian Hospital BMJ supportive. Palliative Care. 2015. doi: 10.1136/bmjspcare-2015-00864

[33] Considine J, et al. Multisite Analysis of Unplanned Transfers [Internet]. Available from: dro.deakin.edu.au/eserv/DU…/considine-multisiteanalysis-2015.pdf [Accessed: January 2017]

[34] Pathan G. recognition and response to the clinically deteriorating patient. Australian Medical Student Journal. 2012. Available from: http://www.amsj.org/archives/2021 [Accessed: November 2016]

[35] Dunning T, Martin P, Savage S, Duggan N. Guidelines for Managing Diabetes at the End of Life [Internet]. 2010. http://www.adma.org.au/clearinghouse/doc_details/35-guidelines-for-managing-diabetes-at-the-end of-life.html [Accessed: December 2016]

[36] Diabetes UK. End of Life Diabetes Care: A Strategy Document [Internet]. 2012. Available from: https://www.diabetes.org.uk/end-of-life-care [Accessed: February 2016]

[37] Carey M, Shah S, DeWilde S. Increased risk of acute cardiovascular events after partner bereavement. JAMA Internal Medicine. 2014;**174**(4):598-605. DOI:10.1001/jamainternalmed.2013.4558

[38] Family caregiver Alliance. Caregiver Health [Internet]. 2010. Available form: http//:www.caregiver.org/caregiver/jsp/content_node.jsp?nodeid+1822 [Accessed: October 2016]

[39] Buckley T, Sunari D, Marshall A, et al. Physiological correlates of bereavement and the impact of bereavement interventions. Dialogues in Clinical Neuroscience. 2012;**14**(92):129-139

[40] Lynn J, Adamson D. Living Well at the End of Life Adapting Health Care to Serious Chronic Illness in Old Age. Santa Monica RAND, CA: Rand Corporation; 2003

[41] Dunning T. Palliative and end-of-life care – older people with diabetes. Iinnovage. 2016;**14**:6-8

[42] Beckford M. Quality of life more important than length of time left. The Telegraph. 2011. www.telegraph.co.uk/.../Quality-of-life-more-important-than-length-of-time-left.html

[43] Ali N, Chawla J. Failure to thrive in elderly adults. Medscape. 2015 Available from: http://emedicine.medscape.com/article/2096163-overview [Accessed: May 2017]

[44] Berger N, Savvides P, Koroukian S, et al. Cancer in the elderly. American Clinical and Climatological Association. 2006;**117**:147-156

[45] Giovinnucci E, Harlan D, Archer M, Bergenstal R, et al. Diabetes and cancer. Diabetes Care. 2010;**33**(7):1674-1685

[46] Spence Scott P. The Passing: What to Expect When Witnessing a Loved One's Death [Internet]. 2016. Available from: https://www.caring.com/articles/witness-passing-away [Accessed: November 2016]

[47] Kitzelman K, Kent E, Mollica M, Rowland J. How does carer wellbeing relate to perceived quality of life in patients with cancer? Journal Clinical Oncology 2016;**34**:3554-3561. DOI: 10.1200/oco.2016.67.3434

[48] Savage S, Duggan N, Dunning T, Martin P. The experiences and care preferences of people with diabetes at the end of life: A qualitative study. Journal Hospice and Palliative Care Nursing. 2012;**14**(4):293-302

[49] Quinn K, Hudson P, Dunning T. Diabetes management in patients receiving palliative care. Journal Pain and Symptom Management. 2007;**32**(3):275-286

[50] Stolberg C. A Conversation with Dame Cecily Saunders, Reflecting on a Life of Treating Death and Dying [Internet]. 1999. Available from: www.nytimes.com/.../conversation-with-dame-cicely-saunders-reflecting-life-treating-dying.html [Accessed: November 2016]

[51] Australian Diabetes Educators Association (ADEA). Clinical Guiding Principles for Subcutaneous Insulin Injection Technique. Canberra: ADEA; 2017

## Some useful resources

### Position statements

Australian Commission on Safety and Quality in Health Care. National Consensus Statement: Essential Elements for Safety and High-quality End-of-life Care [Internet]. 2015. Available from: www.safetyandquality.gov.au/…/National-Consensus-Statement-Essential-Elements-forsafe-high-quality-end-of-life-care.pdf

Association of British Diabetologists. Position Statement: Diabetes and End-of-Life Care [Internet]. 2011. Available from: www.diabetologists-abcd.org.uk/position_papers.htm

Palliative Care Australia Alzheimer's Australia Palliative Care and Dementia [Internet]. Available from: https://www.fightdementia.org.au/…/20130905_PCA_Alzheimerpositionstatementinfront.pdf

### Guidelines

Diabetes UK. 2013 End of Life Diabetes Care [37].

Dunning T, Martin P, Savage S, Duggan N. Guidelines for Managing Diabetes at the End of Life [Internet]. 2010. http://www.adma.org.au/clearinghouse/doc_details/35-guidelines-for-managing-diabetes-at-the-end of-life.html [35].

Dunning T, Savage S, Duggan N. The McKellar Guidelines for Managing Older People with Diabetes in Residential and Other Care Settings [Internet]. 2013. Available from: www.adma.org.au/…/133-the-mckellar-guidelines-for-managing-older-people-with-diabetes-in-residential-and-other-care-settings_9dec2013 [15].

International Diabetes' Federation (IDF). Global Guideline for Managing Older People with Type 2 Diabetes [Internet]. 2013. Available from: www.idf.org [3].

### Other publications

Sweriessen H, Duckett S. Dying well: The Grattan Report. 2014. ISBN: 1-925015-81-4 [30].

Gold Standards Framework Centre. Prognostic Indicator Guidance [Internet]. 2011. Available from: http://www.goldstandardsframework.org.uk/cd-contemt/uploads/files/General%Files/Prognostic%20Indicator%20Guidance%20October%201011.pdf [31].

American Academy hospice and Palliative Medicine, Palliative Care Medicine, Centre to Advance palliative Care, Hospice and Palliative Care Nurses Association, Last Act partnership. National consensus project for quality palliative care: clinical practice guidelines for quality palliative care: Executive summary. Journal Palliative Medicine. 2004;**5**:611-627

Section 4

# Prognostic Models in Palliative Care

Chapter 7

# Prognosis Prediction Models and their Clinical Utility in Palliative Care

Yu Uneno and Masashi Kanai

Additional information is available at the end of the chapter

http://dx.doi.org/10.5772/intechopen.69663

**Abstract**

Prognosis prediction is a clinically relevant issue to facilitate optimal decision-making for both physicians and patients with cancer. Many previous studies revealed that prognosis prediction based on the physician's intuition and/or clinical experience is inaccurate and often optimistic, which means that there is a tendency to overestimate patient survival in daily clinical practice. In recent decades, many efforts have been made to develop prognosis prediction models which aid physicians to make more accurate prognosis prediction. In this chapter, we review the representative prognosis prediction models in palliative care and related studies. In addition, we refer to several prognosis prediction models developed by unique methods (for instance, case-crossover design or machine learning). Finally, we focus on the possible clinical utility of prognosis prediction models. In fact, no previous studies have clearly demonstrated whether the application of such prognosis prediction models truly benefits patient care in daily clinical practice. Therefore, we will discuss how the application of prognosis prediction models could benefit patients under palliative care.

**Keywords:** cancer, clinical prediction of survival, clinical utility, palliative care, prognosis prediction model

## 1. Introduction

Prognosis is one of the most relevant concerns for both patients and healthcare professionals (HCPs). Patients with advanced cancer and their families are required to make decisions such as choosing treatment alternatives or place to spend their end of life or that of their family members. In particular, timing in discontinuing palliative chemotherapy largely affects end-of-life care. Continuing ineffective palliative chemotherapy at the end of life increases life-threatening adverse events (AEs), hospital administration associated with AEs, and medical cost [1, 2]. Furthermore, it causes patients' quality of life (QOL) to deteriorate, delays hospice referral, and deprives patients of the chance to die in their preferred place [3, 4]. Thus, optimal prognosis prediction is essential for better end-of-life care.

Subjective prognosis prediction based on HCPs' experience or intuition is a simple method, which requires no special device in daily practice. However, this method is often inaccurate or tends to overestimate patient survival [5]. Therefore, development of more accurate objective prognosis prediction methods is warranted.

In recent decades, several prognosis prediction models have been developed by integrating known prognostic factors [6–8]. These models have been validated in clinical settings across several countries and their accuracy have been compared [9, 10]. Moreover, studies exploiting new prognostic factors, such as phase angle or circadian rhythm, have been reported in Refs. [11, 12].

Recent progress in informatics has enabled us to retrieve and analyze clinical big data comprehensively, and new methods, such as machine learning or artificial intelligence, have been utilized to develop prognosis prediction models [13, 14]. We also review these issues in this chapter.

Finally, we focus on the clinical utility of prognosis prediction models, which has long been beyond the scope of the main issues in this research field.

## 2. Current status of prognosis prediction

### 2.1. Subjective prognosis prediction

Subjective prognosis prediction based on HCPs' experience or intuition is referred to as clinical prediction of survival (CPS). CPS is one of the most classic styles and has long been used in daily clinical practice. CPS utilizes three common questions. The first question is the "temporal" question, asking "how long can the patient live?" The second question is the "surprise" question, asking "will you be surprised if the patient dies within a specific term?" and the third question is the "probabilistic" question, asking "what is the patient's probability of survival within a specific term?"

The temporal question seems to be the most common prediction type in clinical practice. The answer to this question provides clear and simple information to HCPs. However, there are problems in its accuracy. Hui et al. reported its accuracy as just 32% among eight physicians and 18% among 20 nurses [15]. Moreover, 60% of nurses gave an optimistic prediction of survival [15]. Consistent with these results, another group reported that 63% of prognosis prediction estimated by HCPs was optimistic [16].

The surprise question has a feature of higher negative predictive value (NPV), which is more than 90% in two independent studies [17, 18]. Therefore, the surprise question has been used to identify patients who have a limited survival, and answering "no" is thought to signal the ideal time for specific action such as advance care planning (ACP) [19].

The probabilistic question showed a higher accuracy than the temporal question. The accuracy of physicians' prediction of death within 24 and 48 h was 71–73% and 66–67%, respectively [15, 20]. Interestingly, nurses showed more favorable predictive performance than physicians using the probabilistic question, and the accuracy of their prediction of death within 24 h and 48 h was 90–91% and 83–86%, respectively [15, 20].

### 2.2. Objective prognosis prediction

As discussed in Section 2.1, each CPS may have promising performance in specific settings; however, their accuracy is not satisfactory and is often optimistic [5, 16, 21]. To cope with these problems, many efforts have been made to develop more accurate prognosis prediction models using known prognostic factors.

#### *2.2.1. Prognostic factors*

Prognostic factors are classified into two groups, one composed of clinical signs/symptom and the other of laboratory data. Performance status [22–24], dyspnea [25, 26], malnutrition [27, 28], appetite/weight loss [29], and delirium [30, 31] are well-known clinical factors. Recently, novel prognostic factors have been proposed. Phase angle, which is measured via bioelectrical impedance analysis (BIA), reflects the amount of water in tissues (resistance) and cellular membrane (capacitance) and could be a prognostic factor [11]. Circadian rhythm is also found to be an independent prognostic factor [12, 32].

Laboratory factors include inflammatory markers (for instance, C-reactive protein (CRP), erythrocyte sedimentation, or neutrophil lymphocyte ratio) [33, 34], nutrition markers (for instance, albumin) [35, 36], and tumor progression markers (for instance, calcium or lactate dehydrogenase) [37, 38].

#### *2.2.2. Prognosis prediction model*

In recent decades, many prognostic models have been developed integrating a variety of prognostic factors, CPS, and other patients' information, and their accuracy is improving.

When we use these models in practice, we need to pay attention to the fitness of prediction models for treating patients. In other words, we should verify the clinical settings under which the prediction model was developed. When the clinical settings for treating patients are similar to those of the original study, the prognostic model may fit that patient; otherwise, we should exercise caution when applying prognostic models.

We reviewed the previously proposed prognostic models in the palliative care setting as shown below and summarized the characteristics of each model in **Table 1**.

##### *2.2.2.1. The palliative prognostic index (PPI)*

The palliative prognostic index (PPI) is a noninvasive prognostic model developed by Morita et al. in 1999 and requires no laboratory items (**Table 1**) [6].

| Model | Items | Risk groups |
|---|---|---|
| Palliative prognostic index [6] | Palliative prognostic index (0–4 points)<br>Oral intake (0–2.5 points)<br>Edema (0, 1 point)<br>Dyspnea at rest (0, 3.5 points)<br>Delirium (0, 4 points) | (A) Median survival 155 days: PPI ≤ 2.0<br>(B) Median survival 89 days: 2.0 < PPI ≤ 4.0<br>(C) Median survival 18 days: 4.0 < PPI |
| Palliative prognostic score [7] | Dyspnea (0, 1 point)<br>Anorexia (0, 1.5 points)<br>Karnofsky performance scale ≥ 50% (0, 2.5 points)<br>Clinical prediction of survival (0–8.5 points)<br>Total white blood cell (0–1.5 points)<br>Lymphocyte percentage (0–2.5 points) | (A) 30-Day survival probability > 70%, 0–5.5 points<br>(B) 30-Day survival probability 30–70%, 5.6–11.0 points<br>(C) 30-Day survival probability < 30%, 11.1–17.5 points |
| Glasgow prognostic score [62] | C-Reactive protein<br>Albumin | Score 0: C-Reactive protein ≥ 10 mg/l and albumin ≥ 35g/l<br>Score 1: C-reactive protein > 10 mg/l or albumin < 35 g/l<br>Score 2: C-reactive protein >10 mg/l and albumin < 35 g/l |
| Prognosis in palliative care study predictor models A [8] | Mental test score >3<br>Pulse rate<br>Presence of distant metastasis<br>Site of metastases (liver)<br>ECOG score<br>Global health score<br>Loss of appetite<br>Site of metastases (bone)<br>Difficulty in breathing<br>Difficulty in swallowing<br>Primary breast cancer<br>Primary male genital cancer (including prostate)<br>Weight loss | Days: <14 days<br>Weeks: 14–55 days<br>Months+: >55 days<br>*See detail in "THE PiPS PROGNOSTICATOR" |
| Prognosis in palliative care study predictor models B [8] | Pulse rate<br>White blood count<br>Platelets<br>Urea<br>C-Reactive protein<br>Global health score<br>Alanine transaminase<br>Mental test score >3<br>Distant metastasis<br>Site of metastases (bone)<br>Lack of appetite<br>ECOG score<br>Neutrophils<br>Lymphocytes<br>Alkaline phosphatase<br>Albumin<br>Primary male genital cancer (including prostate)<br>Tired | Days: <14 days<br>Weeks: 14–55 days<br>Months+: >55 days<br>*See detail in "THE PiPS PROGNOSTICATOR" |

*THE PiPS PROGNOSTICATOR: http://www.pips.sgul.ac.uk/.

**Table 1.** Representative prognosis prediction models in palliative care.

Validation studies of the PPI were performed in Japan, Taiwan, Kuwait, Ireland, the United Kingdom, and Australia [39–46]. Morita et al. revealed that the PPI significantly reduced overestimation of survival compared to the CPS [39]. In the study of another group, the PPI was assessed by a nurse specialist, and the area under the curve (AUC) of the receiver operating characteristic (ROC) to predict death within 21 days was 0.68 [40]. In Kuwait, Alshemmari et al. revealed that the PPI can be a helpful tool in predicting hospital mortality of patients with advanced cancer in an acute care setting and that the hospital mortality rate for patients with a PPI score ≥ 6 was significantly higher than for those with a PPI score < 6 (93% versus 56% $p < 0.001$) [41].

In addition to the validation studies, studies which aimed to modify PPI were also reported. Two modified PPI models were tested in sub-analysis of the Japan-prognostic assessment tools validation (J-ProVal) study. The one substitutes the Communication Capacity Scale (CCS) for delirium to the required items of PPI [47]. The other adds a new item about the activities of daily living changes to the PPI; however, this did not significantly improve its prognostic value [48].

Moreover, some researchers examined the longitudinal score change of the PPI [49, 50].

#### 2.2.2.2. *Palliative prognostic (PaP) score*

In 1999, Pirovano et al. proposed the palliative prognostic (PaP) score (**Table 1**) [7]. In this prospective cohort study, 519 patients with advanced cancer were recruited at 22 institutions in Italy, and a scoring model with a range of 0–17.5 points was developed. The score was able to subdivide the population into three risk groups [7]. The PaP score has been validated in both oncological and palliative settings.

In the palliative setting, the validation studies were performed in Australia, Italy, Brazil, and Canada [51–55]. Glare and Virik prospectively recruited 100 consecutive patients referred to palliative medicine consultative services. In this study, each of the three risk groups showed significantly different median survivals (60, 34, and 8 d, respectively) [51].

In the oncology setting, the validation studies were performed in Australia, Italy, and Japan [56–59]. Initially, a validation study of the oncology setting was reported by Glare et al. in 2004, recruiting 100 patients receiving medical or radiation oncology care [56]. The median survival of three risk groups was 17, 7, and < 1 w, respectively. A retrospective study of Ikeguchi et al. was unique because it revealed that patients with non-resectable gastric cancer who were classified into the low-risk group by the PaP score received a more toxic first-line regimen, whereas patients with a high-risk score received a less toxic regimen [57]. Ikeguchi et al. concluded that the PaP score may be a promising tool for selecting a chemotherapy regimen for patients with non-resectable gastric cancer.

Studies modifying the PaP score are also reported. In 2011, Scarpi et al. proposed the D-PaP score, which added the item of delirium into the PaP score [60]. Interestingly, Hui et al. revealed that the PaP score without the CPS showed a better predictive performance than the original PaP score in 2016 [61]. This suggested that the addition of the CPS to the PaP score may actually reduce its accuracy. Further comparison of the PaP score with or without the CPS would be of value.

#### 2.2.2.3. Glasgow prognostic score (GPS)

The Glasgow prognostic score (GPS) is a simple prognostic model based on inflammatory markers, which requires only a CRP and albumin (**Table 1**). The GPS is a prognostic model with the most abundant evidence, and more than 60 papers recruiting more than 30,000 participants have been reported in Ref. [62].

However, studies of the GPS in a palliative care setting are scare. Partridge et al. retrospectively examined the prognostic performance of 120 patients with advanced cancer at a single institution in the United Kingdom [63]. In this study, patients with a modified GPS of 2 had 2.7 times higher risk of death compared to those with a modified GPS of 0 [63]. In the J-ProVal study, Miura et al. prospectively recruited 1160 patients in palliative care settings [64]. They reported that the positive predictive value (PPV) and NPV of 6 weeks of prognosis of patients with a GPS of 2 were 0.733 and 0.611, respectively.

#### 2.2.2.4. Prognosis in palliative care study (PiPS) predictor model

In 2011, Gwilliam et al. proposed the prognosis in palliative care study (PiPS) model (**Table 1**). In this prospective cohort study, 1018 patients with cancer were recruited from 18 institutions in the United Kingdom [8]. The PiPS-A model does not require laboratory items and showed an AUC of 0.79. The PiPS-B model requires laboratory items and showed an AUC of 0.86.

Since the PiPS model is a relatively newer prognostic model, the number of validation studies is limited [65, 66]. In 2015, Kim et al. reported a validation study of 202 patients with advanced cancer at the palliative care unit (PCU) in Korea [65]. Both the PiPS-A model and the PiPS-B model effectively predicted median survival in the "days" and "weeks" groups; however, it did not in the "months" group [65]. Further validation of the PiPS model is warranted.

### 2.2.3. Comparison among prognosis prediction models

Direct comparison of different prognostic models in the same cohort is important, because it indicates the usefulness and appropriate clinical use of each model. There are some comparative studies [9, 43, 67], and the largest is the J-ProVal study reported by Baba et al.

Baba et al. tested five different prognosis models: the PaP score, the D-PaP score, the PPI model, the PiPS-A model, and the PiPS-B model [10]. Concerning feasibility, prognostic models without laboratory tests (the PPI model and the PiPS-A model) showed more than 90% feasibility in all palliative care settings, including home care services. Meanwhile, the feasibility of the PaP score, the D-PaP score, and the PiPS-B model, all of which require laboratory items, was 60–80%. In particular, the feasibility of home palliative care services was only 30–40%. Concerning predictive value, the PPI showed a significantly lower C-index than the PaP score and the D-PaP score in almost all settings. The modified PiPS model showed equivalent or superior accuracy to the PaP score and the D-PaP score in all settings [10]. The authors concluded that the "PPI is simple and highly feasible, and seems to be suitable for routine clinical use for situations where rough estimates of prognosis are sufficient and/or patients do not want invasive procedures. Although the PiPS-A model requires 13 items, it provides higher predictive value without invasive procedure.

If laboratory items are available, the PaP score, D-PaP score and PiPS-B model would be more appropriate" [10].

*2.2.4. Other prognosis prediction models*

In addition to the abovementioned representative prognostic models, other prognostic models are proposed, including the indicator of poor prognosis [68], the Vitamin B12/CRP index [69, 70], the terminal cancer prognostic score [71], the Chuang prognostic score [72, 73], the prognostic 7-day survival formula [74], the Chinese prognostic scale [75], the computer-assisted model [76], the Japan palliative oncology study-prognostic index [77], the objective prognostic score [78, 79], the prognostic nomogram for terminally ill cancer patients [80], and the symptom-based predictive tool [81]. Further validation studies or comparative studies among those models are warranted.

*2.2.5. Novel research fields of prognosis prediction models*

*2.2.5.1. Prediction of sudden unexpected death (SUD)*

Prediction of sudden unexpected death (SUD) is a novel and pivotal research field. SUD has no clear definition, but it is often recognized as sudden death that occurs earlier than anticipated [82, 83]. Prevalence of SUD ranges between 0.5 and 23% in the palliative care setting [82]. SUD shows no impending death sign, such as nonreactive pupils, decreased urine output, and peripheral cyanosis, which makes SUD more difficult to predict [82]. Meanwhile, SUD exposes patients, caregivers, and HCPs to serious burden [84]. Particularly, SUD is significantly associated with depression, panic disorder, alcohol use disorder, or social isolation for caregivers or bereaved families [85, 86]. Thus, identifying factors relating to the occurrence of SUD is richly warranted.

*2.2.6. Prognosis prediction model using machine learning techniques or artificial intelligence*

Because of the progress in the field of informatics, big data can be managed more easily and promptly than ever before. Correspondingly, the number of publications applying novel informatics techniques is rising in clinical research. Prognosis prediction models using machine learning techniques or artificial intelligence have been proposed in the oncology setting [13, 14]. In the coming decades, multidisciplinary studies featuring collaborations between informatics specialists and HCPs are likely to be accelerated. In the palliative care setting, since invasive procedures are generally avoided, the amount of available clinical data—such as blood tests or imaging tests—is limited. This may cause delays in the progress of informatics in the palliative care setting. Therefore, improving data retrieving systems, including those subjective clinical symptoms recorded in text style (for instance, pain, nausea, and appetite loss), will play a key role in the progress of palliative care research.

## 3. Future plan

Many efforts, reviewed in this chapter, have been made toward developing prognostic models and improving their accuracy. We are also developing a novel prognosis prediction model, which is "adaptable." Conventional prognostic models are developed using the data obtained from a single time point (for instance, a baseline assessment date). This study design limits the use of these models under baseline conditions. Because patients' condition during treatment course can change from the baseline, development of an adaptable prognosis prediction model, which could be applied at any time point after the initiation of chemotherapy, is warranted in practice. Thus, we are developing adaptable prognostic models for patients with cancer receiving chemotherapy [87]. In this case-crossover study, we recruited 2693 patients, and 3,471,521 laboratory data at 115,738 time points, representing 40 laboratory items that were monitored for 1 year before the death event, were applied in developing prognostic models. The prognosis prediction model utilizing albumin, lactate dehydrogenase, and neutrophils was selected based on its strong ability to predict death events within 1 month–6 months, and the AUC for 1-month and 2-month models was more than 0.80. We plan to compare this novel model with existing conventional models.

Meanwhile, apart from the effort to predict more accurate prognosis, we should also focus on the issue that no previous studies clearly demonstrated whether application of such prognosis prediction models truly benefits patient care in daily clinical practice. There are concerns that we may be satisfied merely with developing or using prognosis prediction models but pay less attention to assessing their clinical utility. Next, we consider how prognosis prediction can benefit patients.

### 3.1. Efficacy of prognosis prediction for cancer patients

#### *3.1.1. Clinical utility of prognostic disclosure*

First, how many patients are willing to have their prognosis disclosed to them? Although it differs across studies, the proportion is reported to be 40–60% [88, 89]. It was shown that patients were willing to know their life expectancy in greater detail than anticipated by HCPs [90]. Thus, HCPs need to disclose the prognosis properly to patients who want this information.

Studies investigating the clinical outcome of prognostic disclosure are scarce. To the best of our knowledge, there are no clinical trials, but a few observational studies have been reported. In 2015, Enzinger et al. reported on a large prospective cohort study, "Coping with Cancer" [91]. In this study, 590 patients with advanced cancer were analyzed, and patients for whom their prognosis was disclosed had a more realistic understanding of life expectancy than those for whom it was not (median patient self-estimates of life expectancy 12 months versus 48 months). Moreover, patients with a realistic understanding of life expectancy preferred comfort-oriented over life-prolonging care, with a higher likelihood of a do-not-resuscitate order without deteriorating the patients' emotional well-being or the patient-physician relationship [91]. Despite the limitation of being an observational study, however, this study produced meaningful findings for the association between prognosis disclosure and advance care planning (ACP).

Many studies have investigated whether ACP benefited end-of-life management. In the "Coping with Cancer" study, Wright et al. showed that end-of-life discussion was significantly associated with a less aggressive medical care (such as ventilation, ICU admission, and resuscitation), a reduction in the bereaved caregiver's grief or depression, and a longer hospice stay [92]. Other similar studies also showed consistent results [1, 93, 94].

#### 3.1.2. *Clinical utility of prognosis prediction model*

The outcomes of prognosis disclosure based on prognostic models would be expected to be the same as the outcomes referred to in Section 3.1.1. Considering study design is a challenging issue. For example, prognosis disclosure based on prognostic models versus the CPS may be interesting, but it may also introduce some ethical issues that need to be resolved. We hope that the number of studies investigating the clinical utility of prognostic models will increase in the near future.

## 4. Conclusion

A number of prognosis prediction models are proposed, and their accuracy is approaching 80–90%. Novel techniques, such as machine learning or artificial intelligence, would accelerate progress. At the same time, we need to put greater efforts to clarify the clinical utility of prognosis prediction models for patients with cancer, a topic that has been beyond the scope of the main issues in this research field for a long time.

## Author details

Yu Uneno[1] and Masashi Kanai[2*]

*Address all correspondence to: kanai@kuhp.kyoto-u.ac.jp

1 Department of Therapeutic Oncology, Graduate School of Medicine, Kyoto University, Kyoto, Japan

2 Department of Clinical Oncology, Pharmacogenomics and Palliative Medicine, Graduate School of Medicine, Kyoto University, Kyoto, Japan

## References

[1] Wright AA, Zhang B, Keating NL, Weeks JC, Prigerson HG. Associations between palliative chemotherapy and adult cancer patients' end-of-life care and place of death: Prospective cohort study. BMJ 2014;**348**:g1219. DOI: 10.1136/bmj.g1219

[2] Cheung MC, Earle CC, Rangrej J, Ho TH, Liu N, Barbera L, et al. Impact of aggressive management and palliative care on cancer costs in the final month of life. Cancer. 2015;**121**(18):3307-15.

[3] Prigerson HG, Bao Y, Shah MA, Paulk ME, LeBlanc TW, Schneider BJ, et al. Chemotherapy use, performance status, and quality of life at the end of life. JAMA Oncology. 2015;**1**(6): 778-784. DOI: 10.1001/jamaoncol.2015.2378

[4] Wu CC, Hsu TW, Chang CM, Lee CH, Huang CY, Lee CC. Palliative chemotherapy affects aggressiveness of end-of-life care. The Oncologist. 2016;**21**(6):771-777. DOI: 10.1634/theoncologist.2015-0445

[5] Glare P, Virik K, Jones M, Hudson M, Eychmuller S, Simes J, et al. A systematic review of physicians' survival predictions in terminally ill cancer patients. BMJ. 2003;**327**(7408): 195-198. DOI: 10.1136/bmj.327.7408.195

[6] Morita T, Tsunoda J, Inoue S, Chihara S. The Palliative Prognostic Index: A scoring system for survival prediction of terminally ill cancer patients. Supportive Care in Cancer: Official Journal of the Multinational Association of Supportive Care in Cancer. 1999;**7**(3):128-133

[7] Pirovano M, Maltoni M, Nanni O, Marinari M, Indelli M, Zaninetta G, et al. A new palliative prognostic score: A first step for the staging of terminally ill cancer patients. Italian Multicenter and Study Group on Palliative Care. Journal of Pain and Symptom Management. 1999;**17**(4):231-239

[8] Gwilliam B, Keeley V, Todd C, Gittins M, Roberts C, Kelly L, et al. Development of prognosis in palliative care study (PiPS) predictor models to improve prognostication in advanced cancer: Prospective cohort study. BMJ. 2011;**343**:d4920. DOI: 10.1136/bmj.d4920

[9] Maltoni M, Scarpi E, Pittureri C, Martini F, Montanari L, Amaducci E, et al. Prospective comparison of prognostic scores in palliative care cancer populations. The Oncologist. 2012;**17**(3):446-454. DOI: 10.1634/theoncologist.2011-0397

[10] Baba M, Maeda I, Morita T, Inoue S, Ikenaga M, Matsumoto Y, et al. Survival prediction for advanced cancer patients in the real world: A comparison of the Palliative Prognostic Score, Delirium-Palliative Prognostic Score, Palliative Prognostic Index and modified Prognosis in Palliative Care Study predictor model. European Journal of Cancer. 2015;**51**(12):1618-1629. DOI: 10.1016/j.ejca.2015.04.025

[11] Grundmann O, Yoon SL, Williams JJ. The value of bioelectrical impedance analysis and phase angle in the evaluation of malnutrition and quality of life in cancer patients–A comprehensive review. European Journal of Clinical Nutrition. 2015;**69**(12):1290-1297. DOI: 10.1038/ejcn.2015.126

[12] Innominato PF, Focan C, Gorlia T, Moreau T, Garufi C, Waterhouse J, et al. Circadian rhythm in rest and activity: A biological correlate of quality of life and a predictor of survival in patients with metastatic colorectal cancer. Cancer Research. 2009;**69**(11):4700-4707. DOI: 10.1158/0008-5472.can-08-4747

[13] Kourou K, Exarchos TP, Exarchos KP, Karamouzis MV, Fotiadis DI. Machine learning applications in cancer prognosis and prediction. Computational and Structural Biotechnology Journal. 2015;**13**:8-17. DOI: 10.1016/j.csbj.2014.11.005

[14] Enshaei A, Robson CN, Edmondson RJ. Artificial intelligence systems as prognostic and predictive tools in ovarian cancer. Annals of Surgical Oncology. 2015;**22**(12):3970-3975. DOI: 10.1245/s10434-015-4475-6

[15] Hui D, Kilgore K, Nguyen L, Hall S, Fajardo J, Cox-Miller TP, et al. The accuracy of probabilistic versus temporal clinician prediction of survival for patients with advanced cancer: A preliminary report. The Oncologist. 2011;**16**(11):1642-1648. DOI: 10.1634/theoncologist.2011-0173

[16] Christakis NA, Lamont EB. Extent and determinants of error in doctors' prognoses in terminally ill patients: Prospective cohort study. BMJ. 2000;**320**(7233):469-472

[17] Moss AH, Lunney JR, Culp S, Auber M, Kurian S, Rogers J, et al. Prognostic significance of the "surprise" question in cancer patients. Journal of Palliative Medicine. 2010;**13**(7):837-840. DOI: 10.1089/jpm.2010.0018

[18] Hamano J, Morita T, Inoue S, Ikenaga M, Matsumoto Y, Sekine R, et al. Surprise questions for survival prediction in patients with advanced cancer: A multicenter prospective cohort study. The Oncologist. 2015;**20**(7):839-844. DOI: 10.1634/theoncologist.2015-0015

[19] Elliott M, Nicholson C. A qualitative study exploring use of the surprise question in the care of older people: Perceptions of general practitioners and challenges for practice. BMJ Support Palliat Care. 2017;**7**(1):32-38. DOI: 10.1136/bmjspcare-2014-000679

[20] Perez-Cruz PE, Dos Santos R, Silva TB, Crovador CS, Nascimento MS, Hall S, et al. Longitudinal temporal and probabilistic prediction of survival in a cohort of patients with advanced cancer. Journal of Pain and Symptom Management. 2014;**48**(5):875-882. DOI: 10.1016/j.jpainsymman.2014.02.007

[21] Amano K, Maeda I, Shimoyama S, Shinjo T, Shirayama H, Yamada T, et al. The accuracy of physicians' clinical predictions of survival in patients with advanced cancer. Journal of Pain and Symptom Management. 2015;**50**(2):139-146.e1. DOI: 10.1016/j.jpainsymman.2015.03.004

[22] Seow H, Barbera L, Sutradhar R, Howell D, Dudgeon D, Atzema C, et al. Trajectory of performance status and symptom scores for patients with cancer during the last six months of life. Journal of Clinical Oncology. 2011;**29**(9):1151-1158. DOI: 10.1200/jco.2010.30.7173

[23] Downing M, Lau F, Lesperance M, Karlson N, Shaw J, Kuziemsky C, et al. Meta-analysis of survival prediction with Palliative Performance Scale. Journal of Palliative Care. 2007;**23**(4):245-252; discussion 52-4

[24] Myers J, Kim A, Flanagan J, Selby D. Palliative performance scale and survival among outpatients with advanced cancer. Supportive Care in Cancer: Official Journal of the Multinational Association of Supportive Care in Cancer. 2015;**23**(4):913-918. DOI: 10.1007/s00520-014-2440-8

[25] Vigano A, Dorgan M, Buckingham J, Bruera E, Suarez-Almazor ME. Survival prediction in terminal cancer patients: A systematic review of the medical literature. Palliative Medicine. 2000;**14**(5):363-374

[26] Gripp S, Moeller S, Bolke E, Schmitt G, Matuschek C, Asgari S, et al. Survival prediction in terminally ill cancer patients by clinical estimates, laboratory tests, and self-rated anxiety and depression. Journal of Clinical Oncology. 2007;**25**(22):3313-3320. DOI: 10.1200/jco.2006.10.5411

[27] Thoresen L, Frykholm G, Lydersen S, Ulveland H, Baracos V, Prado CM, et al. Nutritional status, cachexia and survival in patients with advanced colorectal carcinoma. Different assessment criteria for nutritional status provide unequal results. Clinical Nutrition (Edinburgh, Scotland). 2013;**32**(1):65-72. DOI: 10.1016/j.clnu.2012.05.009

[28] Tan CS, Read JA, Phan VH, Beale PJ, Peat JK, Clarke SJ. The relationship between nutritional status, inflammatory markers and survival in patients with advanced cancer: A prospective cohort study. Supportive Care in Cancer: Official Journal of the Multinational Association of Supportive Care in Cancer. 2015;**23**(2):385-391. DOI: 10.1007/s00520-014-2385-y

[29] Martin L, Senesse P, Gioulbasanis I, Antoun S, Bozzetti F, Deans C, et al. Diagnostic criteria for the classification of cancer-associated weight loss. Journal of Clinical Oncology. 2015;**33**(1):90-99. DOI: 10.1200/jco.2014.56.1894

[30] Caraceni A, Nanni O, Maltoni M, Piva L, Indelli M, Arnoldi E, et al. Impact of delirium on the short term prognosis of advanced cancer patients. Italian Multicenter Study Group on Palliative Care. Cancer. 2000;**89**(5):1145-1149

[31] Lawlor PG, Gagnon B, Mancini IL, Pereira JL, Hanson J, Suarez-Almazor ME, et al. Occurrence, causes, and outcome of delirium in patients with advanced cancer: A prospective study. Archives of Internal Medicine. 2000;**160**(6):786-794

[32] Levi F, Dugue PA, Innominato P, Karaboue A, Dispersyn G, Parganiha A, et al. Wrist actimetry circadian rhythm as a robust predictor of colorectal cancer patients survival. Chronobiology International. 2014;**31**(8):891-900. DOI: 10.3109/07420528.2014.924523

[33] Maltoni M, Caraceni A, Brunelli C, Broeckaert B, Christakis N, Eychmueller S, et al. Prognostic factors in advanced cancer patients: Evidence-based clinical recommendations—A study by the Steering Committee of the European Association for Palliative Care. Journal of Clinical Oncology. 2005;**23**(25):6240-6248. DOI: 10.1200/jco.2005.06.866

[34] Templeton AJ, McNamara MG, Seruga B, Vera-Badillo FE, Aneja P, Ocana A, et al. Prognostic role of neutrophil-to-lymphocyte ratio in solid tumors: A systematic review and meta-analysis. Journal of the National Cancer Institute. 2014;**106**(6):dju124. DOI: 10.1093/jnci/dju124

[35] Barbot AC, Mussault P, Ingrand P, Tourani JM. Assessing 2-month clinical prognosis in hospitalized patients with advanced solid tumors. Journal of Clinical Oncology. 2008;**26**(15):2538-2543. DOI: 10.1200/jco.2007.14.9518

[36] Vigano A, Bruera E, Jhangri GS, Newman SC, Fields AL, Suarez-Almazor ME. Clinical survival predictors in patients with advanced cancer. Archives of Internal Medicine. 2000;**160**(6):861-868

[37] Donovan PJ, Achong N, Griffin K, Galligan J, Pretorius CJ, McLeod DS. PTHrP-mediated hypercalcemia: Causes and survival in 138 patients. The Journal of Clinical Endocrinology and Metabolism. 2015;**100**(5):2024-2029. DOI: 10.1210/jc.2014-4250

[38] Suh SY, Ahn HY. Lactate dehydrogenase as a prognostic factor for survival time of terminally ill cancer patients: A preliminary study. European Journal of Cancer. 2007;**43**(6):1051-1059. DOI: 10.1016/j.ejca.2007.01.031

[39] Morita T, Tsunoda J, Inoue S, Chihara S. Improved accuracy of physicians' survival prediction for terminally ill cancer patients using the Palliative Prognostic Index. Palliative Medicine. 2001;**15**(5):419-424

[40] Cheng WH, Kao CY, Hung YS, Su PJ, Hsieh CH, Chen JS, et al. Validation of a palliative prognostic index to predict life expectancy for terminally ill cancer patients in a hospice consultation setting in Taiwan. Asian Pacific Journal of Cancer Prevention: APJCP. 2012;**13**(6):2861-2866

[41] Alshemmari S, Ezzat H, Samir Z, Refaat S, Alsirafy SA. The palliative prognostic index for the prediction of survival and in-hospital mortality of patients with advanced cancer in Kuwait. Journal of Palliative Medicine. 2012;**15**(2):200-204. DOI: 10.1089/jpm.2011.0253

[42] Sonoda H, Yamaguchi T, Matsumoto M, Hisahara K. Validation of the palliative prognostic index and palliative prognostic score in a palliative care consultation team setting for patients with advanced cancers in an acute care hospital in Japan. The American Journal of Hospice & Palliative Care. 2014;**31**(7):730-734. DOI: 10.1177/1049909113506034

[43] Chou WC, Kao CY, Wang PN, Chang H, Wang HM, Chang PH, et al. The application of the Palliative Prognostic Index, Charlson comorbidity index, and Glasgow Prognostic Score in predicting the life expectancy of patients with hematologic malignancies under palliative care. BMC Palliative Care. 2015;**14**:18. DOI: 10.1186/s12904-015-0011-5

[44] Stone CA, Tiernan E, Dooley BA. Prospective validation of the palliative prognostic index in patients with cancer. Journal of Pain and Symptom Management. 2008;**35**(6):617-622. DOI: 10.1016/j.jpainsymman.2007.07.006

[45] Subramaniam S, Thorns A, Ridout M, Thirukkumaran T, Osborne TR. Accuracy of prognosis prediction by PPI in hospice in patients with cancer: A multi-centre prospective study. BMJ Supportive & Palliative Care. 2015;**5**(4):399-404. DOI: 10.1136/bmjspcare-2012-000239rep

[46] Yoong J, Atkin N, Le B. Use of the palliative prognostic index in a palliative care consultation service in Melbourne, Australia. Journal of Pain and Symptom Management. 2010;**39**(1):e2-e4. DOI: 10.1016/j.jpainsymman.2009.08.001

[47] Hamano J, Morita T, Ozawa T, Shishido H, Kawahara M, Aoki S, et al. Validation of the simplified palliative prognostic index using a single item from the communication capacity scale. Journal of Pain and Symptom Management. 2015;**50**(4):542-547.e4. DOI: 10.1016/j.jpainsymman.2015.04.021

[48] Hamano J, Tokuda Y, Kawagoe S, Shinjo T, Shirayama H, Ozawa T, et al. Adding items that assess changes in activities of daily living does not improve the predictive accuracy of the Palliative Prognostic Index. Palliative Medicine 2017;**31**(3):258-266. DOI: 10.1177/0269216316650788

[49] Kao CY, Hung YS, Wang HM, Chen JS, Chin TL, Lu CY, et al. Combination of initial palliative prognostic index and score change provides a better prognostic value for terminally ill cancer patients: A six-year observational cohort study. Journal of Pain and Symptom Management. 2014;**48**(5):804-814. DOI: 10.1016/j.jpainsymman.2013.12.246

[50] Hung CY, Wang HM, Kao CY, Lin YC, Chen JS, Hung YS, et al. Magnitude of score change for the palliative prognostic index for survival prediction in patients with poor prognostic terminal cancer. Supportive Care in Cancer: Official Journal of the Multinational Association of Supportive Care in Cancer. 2014;**22**(10):2725-2731. DOI: 10.1007/s00520-014-2274-4

[51] Glare P, Virik K. Independent prospective validation of the PaP score in terminally ill patients referred to a hospital-based palliative medicine consultation service. Journal of Pain and Symptom Management. 2001;**22**(5):891-898

[52] Maltoni M, Nanni O, Pirovano M, Scarpi E, Indelli M, Martini C, et al. Successful validation of the palliative prognostic score in terminally ill cancer patients. Italian Multicenter Study Group on Palliative Care. Journal of Pain and Symptom Management. 1999;**17**(4):240-247

[53] Naylor C, Cerqueira L, Costa-Paiva LH, Costa JV, Conde DM, Pinto-Neto AM. Survival of women with cancer in palliative care: Use of the palliative prognostic score in a population of Brazilian women. Journal of Pain and Symptom Management. 2010;**39**(1):69-75. DOI: 10.1016/j.jpainsymman.2009.05.020

[54] Tarumi Y, Watanabe SM, Lau F, Yang J, Quan H, Sawchuk L, et al. Evaluation of the Palliative Prognostic Score (PaP) and routinely collected clinical data in prognostication of survival for patients referred to a palliative care consultation service in an acute care hospital. Journal of Pain and Symptom Management. 2011;**42**(3):419-431. DOI: 10.1016/j.jpainsymman.2010.12.013

[55] Mendis R, Soo WK, Zannino D, Michael N, Spruyt O. Multidisciplinary prognostication using the palliative prognostic score in an Australian Cancer Center. Palliative Care. 2015;**9**:7-14. DOI: 10.4137/pcrt.s24411

[56] Glare PA, Eychmueller S, McMahon P. Diagnostic accuracy of the palliative prognostic score in hospitalized patients with advanced cancer. Journal of Clinical Oncology. 2004;**22**(23):4823-4828. DOI: 10.1200/JCO.2004.12.056

[57] Ikeguchi M, Kader A, Yoshimoto M, Takaya S, Watanabe J, Fukumoto Y, et al. Usefulness of palliative prognostic score in the treatment of patients with non-resectable gastric cancer. Molecular and Clinical Oncology. 2013;**1**(2):253-256. DOI: 10.3892/mco.2013.66

[58] Tassinari D, Montanari L, Maltoni M, Ballardini M, Piancastelli A, Musi M, et al. The palliative prognostic score and survival in patients with advanced solid tumors receiving chemotherapy. Supportive Care in Cancer: Official Journal of the Multinational Association of Supportive Care in Cancer. 2008;**16**(4):359-370. DOI: 10.1007/s00520-007-0302-3

[59] Numico G, Occelli M, Russi EG, Silvestris N, Pasero R, Fea E, et al. Survival prediction and frequency of anticancer treatment in cancer patients hospitalized due to acute conditions. Role of clinical parameters and PaP score. Supportive Care in Cancer: Official Journal of the Multinational Association of Supportive Care in Cancer. 2011;**19**(11):1823-1830. DOI: 10.1007/s00520-010-1024-5

[60] Scarpi E, Maltoni M, Miceli R, Mariani L, Caraceni A, Amadori D, et al. Survival prediction for terminally ill cancer patients: Revision of the palliative prognostic score with incorporation of delirium. The Oncologist. 2011;**16**(12):1793-1799. DOI: 10.1634/theoncologist.2011-0130

[61] Hui D, Park M, Liu D, Paiva CE, Suh SY, Morita T, et al. Clinician prediction of survival versus the Palliative Prognostic Score: Which approach is more accurate? European Journal of Cancer. 2016;**64**:89-95. DOI: 10.1016/j.ejca.2016.05.009

[62] McMillan DC. The systemic inflammation-based Glasgow Prognostic Score: A decade of experience in patients with cancer. Cancer Treatment Reviews. 2013;**39**(5):534-540. DOI: 10.1016/j.ctrv.2012.08.003

[63] Partridge M, Fallon M, Bray C, McMillan D, Brown D, Laird B. Prognostication in advanced cancer: A study examining an inflammation-based score. Journal of Pain and Symptom Management. 2012;**44**(2):161-167. DOI: 10.1016/j.jpainsymman.2011.08.013

[64] Miura T, Matsumoto Y, Hama T, Amano K, Tei Y, Kikuchi A, et al. Glasgow prognostic score predicts prognosis for cancer patients in palliative settings: A subanalysis of the Japan-prognostic assessment tools validation (J-ProVal) study. Supportive Care in Cancer: Official Journal of the Multinational Association of Supportive Care in Cancer. 2015;**23**(11):3149-3156. DOI: 10.1007/s00520-015-2693-x

[65] Kim ES, Lee JK, Kim MH, Noh HM, Jin YH. Validation of the prognosis in palliative care study predictor models in terminal cancer patients. Korean Journal of Family Medicine. 2014;**35**(6):283-294. DOI: 10.4082/kjfm.2014.35.6.283

[66] Baba M, Maeda I, Morita T, Hisanaga T, Ishihara T, Iwashita T, et al. Independent validation of the modified prognosis palliative care study predictor models in three palliative care settings. Journal of Pain and Symptom Management. 2015;**49**(5):853-860. DOI: 10.1016/j.jpainsymman.2014.10.010

[67] Stiel S, Bertram L, Neuhaus S, Nauck F, Ostgathe C, Elsner F, et al. Evaluation and comparison of two prognostic scores and the physicians' estimate of survival in terminally ill patients. Supportive Care in Cancer: Official Journal of the Multinational Association of Supportive Care in Cancer. 2010;**18**(1):43-49. DOI: 10.1007/s00520-009-0628-0

[68] Bruera E, Miller MJ, Kuehn N, MacEachern T, Hanson J. Estimate of survival of patients admitted to a palliative care unit: A prospective study. Journal of Pain and Symptom Management. 1992;**7**(2):82-86

[69] Geissbuhler P, Mermillod B, Rapin CH. Elevated serum vitamin B12 levels associated with CRP as a predictive factor of mortality in palliative care cancer patients: A prospective study over five years. Journal of Pain and Symptom Management. 2000;**20**(2):93-103

[70] Kelly L, White S, Stone PC. The B12/CRP index as a simple prognostic indicator in patients with advanced cancer: A confirmatory study. Annals of Oncology: Official Journal of the European Society for Medical Oncology/ESMO. 2007;**18**(8):1395-1399. DOI: 10.1093/annonc/mdm138

[71] Yun YH, Heo DS, Heo BY, Yoo TW, Bae JM, Ahn SH. Development of terminal cancer prognostic score as an index in terminally ill cancer patients. Oncology Reports. 2001;**8**(4):795-800

[72] Chuang RB, Hu WY, Chiu TY, Chen CY. Prediction of survival in terminal cancer patients in Taiwan: Constructing a prognostic scale. Journal of Pain and Symptom Management. 2004;**28**(2):115-122. DOI: 10.1016/j.jpainsymman.2003.11.008

[73] Al-Zahrani AS, El-Kashif AT, Mohammad AA, Elsamany S, Alsirafy SA. Prediction of in-hospital mortality of patients with advanced cancer using the Chuang Prognostic Score. The American Journal of Hospice & Palliative Care. 2013;**30**(7):707-711. DOI: 10.1177/1049909112467362

[74] Chiang JK, Lai NS, Wang MH, Chen SC, Kao YH. A proposed prognostic 7-day survival formula for patients with terminal cancer. BMC Public Health. 2009;**9**:365. DOI: 10.1186/1471-2458-9-365

[75] Lingjun Z, Jing C, Jian L, Wee B, Jijun Z. Prediction of survival time in advanced cancer: A prognostic scale for Chinese patients. Journal of Pain and Symptom Management. 2009;**38**(4):578-586. DOI: 10.1016/j.jpainsymman.2008.12.005

[76] Chiang JK, Cheng YH, Koo M, Kao YH, Chen CY. A computer-assisted model for predicting probability of dying within 7 days of hospice admission in patients with terminal cancer. Japanese Journal of Clinical Oncology. 2010;**40**(5):449-455. DOI: 10.1093/jjco/hyp188

[77] Hyodo I, Morita T, Adachi I, Shima Y, Yoshizawa A, Hiraga K. Development of a predicting tool for survival of terminally ill cancer patients. Japanese Journal of Clinical Oncology. 2010;**40**(5):442-448. DOI: 10.1093/jjco/hyp182

[78] Suh SY, Choi YS, Shim JY, Kim YS, Yeom CH, Kim D, et al. Construction of a new, objective prognostic score for terminally ill cancer patients: A multicenter study. Supportive Care in Cancer: Official Journal of the Multinational Association of Supportive Care in Cancer. 2010;**18**(2):151-157. DOI: 10.1007/s00520-009-0639-x

[79] Yoon SJ, Jung JG, Kim JS, Kim SS, Kim S. Retrospective assessment of objective prognostic score in terminally ill Korean patients with cancer. The American Journal of Hospice & Palliative Care. 2014;**31**(4):435-440. DOI: 10.1177/1049909113492557

[80] Feliu J, Jimenez-Gordo AM, Madero R, Rodriguez-Aizcorbe JR, Espinosa E, Castro J, et al. Development and validation of a prognostic nomogram for terminally ill cancer patients. Journal of the National Cancer Institute. 2011;**103**(21):1613-1620. DOI: 10.1093/jnci/djr388

[81] Nabal M, Bescos M, Barcons M, Torrubia P, Trujillano J, Requena A. New symptom-based predictive tool for survival at seven and thirty days developed by palliative home care teams. Journal of Palliative Medicine. 2014;**17**(10):1158-1163. DOI: 10.1089/jpm.2013.0630

[82] Bruera S, Chisholm G, Dos Santos R, Bruera E, Hui D. Frequency and factors associated with unexpected death in an acute palliative care unit: Expect the unexpected. Journal of Pain and Symptom Management. 2015;**49**(5):822-827. DOI: 10.1016/j.jpainsymman.2014.10.011

[83] Hui D. Unexpected death in palliative care: What to expect when you are not expecting. Current Opinion in Supportive and Palliative Care. 2015;**9**(4):369-374. DOI: 10.1097/spc.0000000000000174

[84] Goodlin SJ, Zhong Z, Lynn J, Teno JM, Fago JP, Desbiens N, et al. Factors associated with use of cardiopulmonary resuscitation in seriously ill hospitalized adults. JAMA. 1999;**282**(24):2333-2339

[85] Burton AM, Haley WE, Small BJ. Bereavement after caregiving or unexpected death: Effects on elderly spouses. Aging & Mental Health. 2006;**10**(3):319-326. DOI: 10.1080/13607860500410045

[86] Keyes KM, Pratt C, Galea S, McLaughlin KA, Koenen KC, Shear MK. The burden of loss: Unexpected death of a loved one and psychiatric disorders across the life course in a national study. The American Journal of Psychiatry. 2014;**171**(8):864-871. DOI: 10.1176/appi.ajp.2014.13081132

[87] U Yu, T Kei, T Akiko, O Kazuya, N Akira, Y Daisuke, et al. Establishment of a terminal prognosis prediction model by applying time series analysis to real-world data. Annals of Oncology. 2015;**26**(Suppl 7):vii79-vii105. DOI: 10.1093/annonc/mdv471.84

[88] Elkin EB, Kim SH, Casper ES, Kissane DW, Schrag D. Desire for information and involvement in treatment decisions: Elderly cancer patients' preferences and their physicians' perceptions. Journal of Clinical Oncology. 2007;**25**(33):5275-5280. DOI: 10.1200/jco.2007.11.1922

[89] Hagerty RG, Butow PN, Ellis PA, Lobb EA, Pendlebury S, Leighl N, et al. Cancer patient preferences for communication of prognosis in the metastatic setting. Journal of Clinical Oncology. 2004;**22**(9):1721-1730. DOI: 10.1200/jco.2004.04.095

[90] Fumis RR, De Camargo B, Del Giglio A. Physician, patient and family attitudes regarding information on prognosis: A Brazilian survey. Annals of Oncology: Official Journal of the European Society for Medical Oncology/ESMO. 2012;**23**(1):205-211. DOI: 10.1093/annonc/mdr049

[91] Enzinger AC, Zhang B, Schrag D, Prigerson HG. Outcomes of prognostic disclosure: Associations with prognostic understanding, distress, and relationship with physician among patients with advanced cancer. Journal of Clinical Oncology. 2015;**33**(32):3809-3816. DOI: 10.1200/JCO.2015.61.9239

[92] Wright AA, Zhang B, Ray A, Mack JW, Trice E, Balboni T, et al. Associations between end-of-life discussions, patient mental health, medical care near death, and caregiver bereavement adjustment. JAMA. 2008;**300**(14):1665-1673. DOI: 10.1001/jama.300.14.1665

[93] Tang ST, Liu TW, Liu LN, Chiu CF, Hsieh RK, Tsai CM. Physician-patient end-of-life care discussions: Correlates and associations with end-of-life care preferences of cancer patients-a cross-sectional survey study. Palliative Medicine. 2014;**28**(10):1222-1230. DOI: 10.1177/0269216314540974

[94] Mack JW, Cronin A, Keating NL, Taback N, Huskamp HA, Malin JL, et al. Associations between end-of-life discussion characteristics and care received near death: A prospective cohort study. Journal of Clinical Oncology. 2012;**30**(35):4387-4395. DOI: 10.1200/jco.2012.43.6055